I0428694

THE "CURE" FOR HEALTH CARE REFORM

HEALTHY WAYS TO HELP ELIMINATE YOUR MEDICAL BILLS

JOAN YORK, B.S.

Copyright © 2011 Joan York B.S.

All rights reserved.

ISBN: 1466477032

ISBN 13: 9781466477032

TABLE OF CONTENTS

FOOD FACTS

ALTERNATIVE HEALTH REMEDIES

MEDICAL ISSUES

PSYCHOLOGICAL STRESS FACTORS

MISCELLANEOUS

CONCLUSION

INTRODUCTION

If you don't think you've been brainwashed regarding your food, see if this sounds familiar. You go to the supermarket where you purchase some healthy food and some food not so healthy, but you justify the non healthy food because it tastes so good and you don't eat it all the time. You have been taught that any disease can strike you or your family at any time. This necessitates a trip to the doctor for drugs or treatment at which point you get better, worse or stay the same, but there is very little you can do to ward off a disease that wants to "get" you.

And for almost every type of ailment there is a corresponding drug to take, whether it is over the counter or prescription.

Imagine a world where disease is rarely a threat to you on any level, and you can live your days with the peace of mind that you will most likely not receive "bad news" from the doctor. If this sounds impossible, the contents of this book will teach you some secrets I've learned over the years.

Here's what you MUST do to get to this point. The key to everything is PREVENTION. First, you need to train yourself to read the labels on the food you eat and substitute the improper food for the "real deal". This will be explained in detail in subsequent chapters. The real food actually will taste better than the tainted stuff available in the stores. It will take a couple of weeks for your taste buds to completely convert to the real food but you'll be amazed at the new wonderful new world of taste.

The formula works something like this - you eat the foods that your body was designed for and disease will have a hard time gaining a foothold. In my late 60's I should be having all sorts of health issues, yet I take absolutely no drugs (they make me sick) and no over the counter remedies If I do develop a mild ailment, I take a natural remedy which works very well instead of popping a pill for every symptom.

As a result, I have a very happy liver that doesn't have to work hard to eliminate drugs and I don't have to deal with the multitude of nasty side effects that the drug manufacturers warn about. It's hard to believe that some drugs have a possible side effect of "death" and that they sell very well. Guess the people who suffered this side effect are not talking.

Taking drugs usually causes your body to object to them by producing a multitude of "side effects". These drugs collect in your liver (not all of them get fully excreted) and frankly, they interfere with the everyday working of your body. Sometime down the road of time the "piper" will be paid.

This key to greatly reducing health expenses may at first sound strange to you, but even though it may seem painful, you won't be giving up eating delicious food, just substituting real food for the counterfeit and harmful ingredients. Eating 'tampered with' food will ultimately cause disease and, more likely than not, a shortened life expectancy. The problem is that it is very hard to directly link a bad diet with one's health problems. If you bite down on a cyanide capsule, you see the effects of this chemical immediately (instant death). Unfortunately, the poisons in our food supply take longer to kill us and it is difficult, if not impossible, to trace our ailments back to the particular food or foods that caused the problem.

I realize there are some of you who will refuse to make any kind of change and that's your prerogative, however, you will still have the same medical situations you started with and the prospect of more illness to come.

But consider this – you wake up in the morning and the poisoning starts with brushing your teeth with a toothpaste with SLS (sodium laurel sulphate, known to have a negative effect on your hormone balance, gender confusion, eye irritation, affects protein structure). You continue with your shower, breathe in its chlorine fumes, (well water does not have this), and have a drink of tap water with its chemicals and carcinogens.

Now it's time for breakfast, cereal that has been refined, milk loaded with antibiotics and hormones, and/or eggs also with antibiotics and hormones, bacon with its carcinogenic nitrates and lots of salt, or a sugary doughnut with white flour. Lunch and dinner are more of the same including meat with hormones and antibiotics, bread with additives too long to list, fruit sprayed with chemicals and pesticides, etc. Has our health care bill reached the trillions yet? MOST OF THE ABOVE ABUSE OF THE HUMAN BODY IS TOTALLY PREVENTABLE.

Introduction

Here is how most people operate regarding their health.. They go about their daily lives trying to eat somewhat sensibly, taking vitamins once in a while if not daily, and pray that the Russian roulette of disease does not land on your doorstep. It's like being a sitting duck in a shooting gallery. And when your unlucky number comes up, you run to the doctor for help and many times it's too late. What a way to live!

May I suggest a proactive alternative which will require a little bit of effort on your part. Over the years most manufacturers of the foods we buy and eat have succumbed to popular opinion to make the food look more attractive. Case in point, most cooking oil has been greatly refined to give it that crystal clear see appearance rather than a more natural cloudy appearance. This is pretty to look at but harmful for the body as the oil is now severely imbalanced by the high heat it is subjected to in its manufacture with most, if not all, of the nutrients taken out.

Also, it is very understandable that consumers want prices to be as low as possible, but it is impossible for most manufacturers to make a wholesome product at a lower cost without it being mass produced. Instead they resort to cheap fillers such as sugar, salt, etc. which play an enormous role in destroying our health.

I can hear it now "health food tastes terrible, I'd rather take my chances". Well you don't have to take any more chances. The purpose of this book is to guide you into happy, healthy, tasty eating, along with the proper vitamins and supplements which are best for your body.

To those who would dare, I offer this challenge. Eat no chemicals for a period of 3 weeks and then sample some of the 'bad stuff'. After the trial period most people will actually be able to taste the poor quality and chemicals in the altered food. Proof positive! Imagine what this 'stuff' is doing to your body. Actually you don't have to imagine - this book will tell you in detail.

A wise man once said "an ounce of prevention is worth a pound of cure".

We live in a very intelligent society and yet when it comes to our health and feeding our bodies the correct foods to maintain optimum health, the vast majority of us haven't much of a clue.

We wouldn't dream of putting the wrong octane gasoline or oil if we own a very expensive car, we take care of the little details. Our bodies are so much more valuable than the most expensive automobile and yet most of us continually abuse it with junk food.

Junk food extends far beyond fast food. Most of it lies in wait in our supermarkets. The sad truth is that it takes some effort to find the foods our bodies were designed for.

Yes, it's all about design. We don't walk around on our hands, we use our feet; we eat food through our mouths, not our nose or ears. Therefore, the reason we have so much illness that requires such extensive health care is that we are eating these highly processed foods.

Changing your lifestyle can help point you in the right direction so that your health care costs can shrink to a fraction of what they are currently.

Make no mistake, the older one gets, the harder it is to keep your body afloat. This is why I rely heavily on whole food vitamins which are a real healthy alternative to prescriptions at a fraction of the cost. The Reference Guide in the back of this book tells you where to purchase these supplements.

God has equipped our bodies with built in mechanisms to fight infection, ward off disease, etc. It's called our immune system and is something we need to keep operating at peak efficiency.

However, our bodies are not equipped to ward off the constant assault of improper food, unclean air and contaminated water. Amazingly, most people pay little or no attention to these things.

To those who won't listen or simply don't care, the results will be obvious sooner or later. Some persons have a stronger constitution (probably a genetic trait). The skeptics are the first to point out that "Uncle Joe" smoked and ate poorly all his life and yet died at the age of 90". I'm guessing this actually happens in less than 1% of the population.

This book's aim is to give you the blueprint for abundant health.

DISCLAIMER

THE FOLLOWING BOOK IS NOT INTENDED AS A SUBSTITUTE FOR MEDICAL CARE AND IS MERELY AN ALTERNATIVE WHEN CONVENTIONAL MEDICINE HAS FAILED.

FOOD FACTS

CHAPTER 1
Acid vs Alkaline

All foods that we eat have either an acid or alkaline effect on our bodies. The acid wastes attack muscles, joints, and organs causing an almost endless list of ailments while the alkaline reaction produces the opposite effect and energizes the body. The organs become very inefficient in an acid environment which makes one susceptible to disease and even organ failure. Before you get to the transplant stage, check your diet. Truly an ounce of prevention is worth a pound of cure.

Drinking soda is one of the quickest ways to make your body more acidic. A non sugar 100% fruit juice drink is much better for the body. Switching over to healthy food and drink will precipitate a cleansing reaction that can make you a little uncomfortable as the toxins are released from your body. Sweating, nausea, diarrhea, and body aching may be part of the process. This is perfectly normal and indicates you are dong something right, not taking a wrong health turn. You may also experience a cold or virus as your body tells these nasty toxins to get lost. The more toxic you are the longer it will take – a few weeks should be maximum at which time you will feel so much better.

Some other acid facts:

Physical exertion produces acid by-products

Jet lag is the result of positive ions that are acid forming. Taking a chlorophyll product will help with this

Viruses, fungi and bacteria can only survive in an acid environment.

Stress can turn our alkaline food acidic

Hostility toward other persons can make us acidic

* * * *

CHAPTER 2
Sugar, Sugar Everywhere

I recently was reading the label of a name brand jam with huge letters on the label "SUGAR FREE". Bear in mind that any ingredient ending in "ose" or "ol" is a sugar. The product contained polydextrose and sucralose which they labeled as an artificial sweetener (research has linked artificial sweeteners to cancer), 2 preservatives as well as 2 dyes. However, poly-destrose and sucrose ARE SUGARS.

As for the addition of dyes, the color of the fruit should be sufficient. Perhaps the fruit is inferior and does not have sufficient color on its own and if health hazards are a consequence of these dyes, well, "so be it" say the manufacturers. Preservatives do not have to be added if the products are marked "Refrigerate after opening".

Manufacturers have put sugars and high fructose corn syrup in bread, frozen entrees of all kinds, scanned vegetables, soups, tomato sauce, every imaginable item even many items at the deli. Why is that? One possible explanation is that the manufacturers know that putting sugar or sugars in their food stimulates an appetite response for more food, especially for more sweets.

I have noticed in particular that when I ingest even a small amount of white flour (it happens when I'm on the road with few options), I almost immediately get a craving for something sweet. Partners in crime are refined white flour and refined white sugar. Any sugar or corn syrup, etc. that is refined acts the same way in the body. In addition to adding those extra pounds, refined products accelerate the aging process because the body has to work very hard to deal with this deficiency.

You have to hunt a little to find food without all the additives that help throw your body out of balance. A health food store is a good place to start. The extra cost balances out because the natural foods are more filling and thereby you eat less.

Sugar:

Sugar causes platelets to stick together, raises triglycerides and can increase the desire for coffee and tobacco. It is also a factor involved with heart disease.

Contributes to tooth decay by decreasing the effectiveness of white blood cells that eat bacteria

Leaches calcium from the body when consumed in soft drinks

Causes the body to release more adrenalin which can be linked to hyper-activity in children and adults

Causes the pancreas to create an abnormal amount of insulin which can lead to diabetes

Becomes an obstacle to weight loss by causing the body to store excess carbohydrates as fat

Can lead to chronic fatigue

Can cause mood swings, anxiety and irritability

Fruit and non sugar fruit juices are wonderful substitutes for the "refined bad stuff". Supermarkets like Shop Rite are starting to come around and offer organic sections, halleluiah!

When sugar is refined, it is transformed from a complex sugar to a simple sugar and when eaten, it causes the body to go into overdrive causing one's blood sugar level elevate very fast. This puts extra strain on the pancreas to regulate this runaway blood sugar level by releasing large amounts of insulin. After years of this abuse, the pancreas wears out and stops producing insulin, thereby creating another diabetic person in our society.

There are approximately 25.8 million adults and children diabetics in the United States, and at least 1 million undetected diabetics, most of which are a direct result of this process. The projected number of diabetics in the US is expected to equal 1/3 of the population in a matter of decades.

As key components of the sugar are removed in the refining process, the end product does not possess all the elements necessary for complete metabolism and digestion, therefore, the brain recognizes this imbalance and signals for more food. Of course the more food one consumes the better the food manufacturers like it. The same is not true for our bodies which can then accumulate excess weight.

Two main offenders are birthdays and Halloween. Both are sugar holidays and hurt people in the name of having fun. Sorry, but that's the way it is.

Unrefined or complex sugars such as raw fruit enter the body slowly at the rate in which they were intended and do not trigger insulin levels to rise unchecked.

While it is true that corn sugar and cane sugars are the same, the key is whether or not they are refined. BECAUSE THEY ARE ALTERED REFINED SUGARS HAVE A MAJOR TENDENCY TO PUT WEIGHT ON THE BODY BECAUSE THEY ARE IMBALANCED AND BAD FOR YOU. In addition, they act as an appetite stimulant because their imperfect state sends a delayed signal to the brain that the hunger or satiety center is satisfied. The end result is that you ingest more calories than you actually need. The latest statistic is that over 60% of all Americans are overweight. EEK!!! Obesity is responsible for a large number of diseases and medical problems which, in turn, require medical assistance. This costs money either to the individual or the government or both. Getting to the root of the problem through prevention saves everyone time, money, and stress.

Solution – read food labels religiously and avoid foods that end in "ose", "ol" or state "sugar", or "brown sugar" which is actually white sugar with molasses added. Fruit juice sweetened, maple syrup, honey, agave and stevia are much more preferable, but take care not to overdue these foods ad they have a tendency to harbor many calories. A health food store is a good choice to locate these natural foods.

When cooking, stevia, agave, and unrefined sugar granules or crystals work very well.

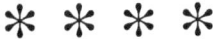

CHAPTER 3
The Hidden Dangers
Of White Flour

Back in the 'old days' and certainly before my time, school children did not have access to the myriad of stationery items available to today's kids.

They had to make their own paste for their arts and crafts projects which consisted of mixing white flour and water. If you don't believe me, try mixing this paste and learn a lesson on just what eating this white flour paste does to you body.

White flour is simply whole grain with most, if not all, of the bran, fiber and nutrients removed. When ingested, it has to steal all missing enzymes, etc. from your body which short changes your body's metabolism. This 'paste' paves the road to extreme constipation unless you are eating a great deal of fiber to balance things out. Chances are you're not!

White flour is everywhere, bread, pasta, prepared foods, etc. it even hides out under the name "wheat flour". This simply means that all a manufacturer has to do to call an ingredient "wheat floor" is to put a pinch of whole wheat flour into white flour.

I'm looking at a box of whole grain pasta. This manufacturer has stated that their product is "51% whole wheat". This is a step in the right direction but the balance of the ingredients is mostly white flour. Now to be perfectly honest 100% whole wheat pasta is somewhat heavy in its taste, but the way around this is to use a spelt or brown rice flour (not rice flour bur brown rice flour). You probably will not notice much of a change in the taste and after a while you won't be able to go back to the 'white stuff'. Your taste buds will convert.

True story – I once had a friend call me and ask my advice on what she could do with reference to her health as she had just tested positive for cervical cancer. For the record I did not tell her to stop seeing her doctor or advise her in any way that would conflict with her medical treatment. I simply told her that it would be very beneficial to her body to stop eating white flour and white sugar. Apparently she took my advice because a month later she called with the news that her next pap smear had tested normal and that there was no trace of the cervical cancer. Halleluiah!!

This advice came too late for me as I had a Class 3 pap on a scale of 1-5, 1 being normal and 5 highly malignant. My first reaction to the doctor's phone call was that he was drinking or that the lab had made a mistake as I was only in my mid thirties. However, a trip to his office confirmed that some of my cervical cells had started to change. The remedy in my case was simply to surgically remove these cells. This was before I knew about enzyme therapy and progesterone cream.

This was my wake up call as prior to this diagnosis I regularly ate white flour and white sugar. Didn't think it was that significant. Well after the surgery and a recovery time that consisted of heavy bleeding every time I moved and being bedridden for around 3 weeks. To date I am 98% white flour free, 95% refined sugar free as the refined stuff sneaks into the most mundane of foods.

I have since learned that the way to protect one's body against female cancers is with a drug free hormone cream which has been shown to balance the female body's hormone levels to the extent it can ward off female cancers. This is discussed in detail in the chapter "For Women Only".

God only knows how much other damage refined products cause. The answer is to have all the manufacturers get on board and give us real unaltered food. And yes, this food does cost somewhat more but that is largely because it is not extensively mass produced. By all rights they should become less expensive as the manufacturers can eliminate the step of removing and stripping the outer grain.

Ezekial and Food For Life companies have come out with breads, english muffins, tortillas, etc. that are made exclusively with sprouted grains. These are very tasty and the healthiest breads and English muffins I know of.

More recommendations in the "Joan's Picks" chapter.

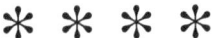

CHAPTER 4
Salt – Just How Bad Is It?

When you start reading food labels and adding up your daily consumption, you'll discover just how much salt you really are ingesting.

The recommended intake is anywhere from 1500 mg. to 2300 mg., use the lower number if you have high blood pressure and/or kidney disease or any other ailment that would suggest you limit your salt intake.

Canned soup is a good example of the salt that manufacturers put in food. Some soup cans contain 2 servings, but the 700-800 mg of salt listed on the can is for ONE serving. Therefore, you must double or multiply the 700-800 by 2 to find out there is 1400-1600 mg. of salt per can. Add this up and you might be taking in 3-4 grams of salt or more on a daily basis from all the foods you ingest. With fast food the amount is usually very high but since there is no label on this food, you would have to ask the establishment to get the exact amount of salt.

SIMPLE RULE OF THUMB – IF YOU OVERWORK A BODY PART OR ORGAN, IT WEARS OUT FASTER and excess salt overworks the heart and kidneys, can lead to a stroke because of unstable blood pressure and can contribute to asthma, Alzheimers, cancer, loss of intelligence and memory. Excess refined salt intake can throw out your salt-potassium balance and lower resistance to illness and disease.

Recently I was out running errands and I felt like I just had to eat something. Here on the East Coast there is very little healthy fast food so I succumbed to a spinach and cheese stromboli. Well, within an hour I started drinking water like a camel, felt very sleepy and groggy, rested a while and started drinking water again 2-3 hours later. This is the body's way of trying to flush out excess salt. Only God and my body knew how much salt was actually in that stromboli, Excess refined salt consumption has been proven to lead to strokes and increase susceptibility to high blood pressure and carcinogens

The sodium that accumulates in the blood holds excess water which makes the heart work heart work harder and increases blood pressure. 2300 mg of salt is the maximum for a healthy adult while 1500 mg is the maximum for an older adult or a person with high blood pressure. Frankly, I think these values are a little high by at least 20%. There are many herb alternatives to flavor one's food. They can be found in the spice section of the supermarket. Unrefined sea salt is a much better alternative but should be used with caution. If your sea salt is pure white, it most likely is refined. Unrefined sea salt is light gray and has all the minerals left untouched.

A corned beef tale – once or twice a year one of the supermarkets I shop at offers a completely natural corned beef with no antibiotics, hormones or preservatives in its own marinade. I have actually looked forward to its arrival. But this year I happened to look at the label more closely and made a shocking discovery. The salt content was 1350 mg per 4 oz. serving. The size of the corned beef was 2.2 lbs for a total of 9 servings. 9 servings times 1350 mg = 12,150 mg salt or MORE THAN 12 GRAMS. It was returned to the store unopened.

This type of food would be good if you really want to encourage kidney failure. The corned beef really had been so delicious that I failed to read the label closely. A word to the wise - this manufacturer has some very good items, but they need to reconsider the amount of salt they put in their foods.

A salt secret – if you are accustomed to eating heavily salted foods, lightly salted food can taste terrible. This is because your taste buds have acclimated to having a lot of salt in and on your food. However, if you cut back on salting your food to the point where you don't need to use much salt, your taste requirement for salt will not require a lot of 'help' from the salt shaker. Using a little of Selina's natural unrefined celtic sea salt from France can actually be beneficial. It may cost more but if you're using less, it really lasts. They have taken salt to a new level with all their flavors. Their salt menu is as follows: celery salt, smoked salt, rosemary salt, toasted sesame salt, toasted garlic salt and original all with 92 minerals. Refined sea salts have almost no minerals. The company also has a book on the subject.

You can also request "no added salt" when ordering at a restaurant – some of the food is prepared in advance and has already been salted, most likely with refined salt, but foods that are cooked to order are at the mercy of the cook's salt shaker.

Please see chapter on "Know Your Serving Sizes".

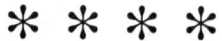

CHAPTER 5
Know Your Serving
Sizes On Labels

Today's manufacturers have resorted to some slight of hand when it comes to serving sizes. For example, some manufacturers list the serving size of their ice cream as ½ cup or four ounces of ice cream. Most people will put much more than 4 oz. in their dish, anywhere from 2-4 times the manufacturers' servings. Now 8 grams of fat per serving translates to 16, 24, or 32 grams of fat in your dish. Heaven forbid you go back for seconds. A 1 ½ quart container contains 12 servings and at 140 calories per serving, this amounts to 1680 calories in addition to 96 grams of fat. No wonder they don't want to put that on the label. 1 1/2 quarts equals ¾ of a half gallon.

Sometimes a frozen food dinner will have 2 servings listed on the label even though the package looks very small. If you are planning on eating the entire amount you must double the calories, sodium, fat etc.

Sodium is another culprit. NACL or sodium chloride, while necessary for the human body, is just not required in the large quantities that are put in our prepared food supply. Case in point, a 7 ½ oz. of canned salmon has

270 mg of salt per serving. This small can is rated at 3 ½ servings or 945 mg of salt. This is almost a full gram (1000 mg).

Canned tomatoes can have 180mg per serving x 3.5 servings = 630 mg of salt for a 14.5 oz can. To make a spaghetti sauce you would probably need 3-4 of these cans or 1890 – 2520 mg. of salt. Dollars to doughnuts the cook will then add additional salt to the mixture. EEK!!!

A 7 oz can of tuna usually contains 750 mg of salt, an 18.8 oz can of premium soup contains 1720 mg salt etc. This excess salt puts an enormous strain on out kidneys and can ultimately lead to kidney failure. Failure of both kidneys without a transplant is a life on dialysis (which can fail) or certain death. The problem is that when we are accustomed to ingesting large amounts of salt, our food tastes bland without it and so the cycle continues as we use more salt. When encountering a food that is heavily salted, I simply can't eat it because my taste buds are in line with what my body requires.

The body reacts to this excess by calling for water to help flush out the salt as it doesn't need this high amount of salt and is trying to excrete it. Have you even eaten fast food and then found you were so very thirsty?

The frozen lasagna story – I had purchased a different brand frozen lasagna and one night I heated it up and proceeded to eat it. After a few minutes of eating this normal size lasagna I was hit with this incredible thirst bomb, the Sahara Desert literally came to mind. After drinking a glass of water I ran for the lasagna box to see just how much salt was in this dinner. First of all, the box read 2.5 servings, followed by 960 mg of salt per serving for a whopping total of 2400 mg of salt, nearly 2 ½ grams. In my opinion, this is a form of low level poisoning – too much refined salt can literally kill you (the natural sea salts are much safer). In addition the label that listed the sodium, fat, etc., was in print that was half the normal size. This product would taste just as good, if not better, with less than half the amount of sodium.

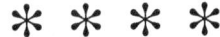

CHAPTER 6
Caffeine – The Mean Bean
Everything You Don't
Want To Know

Caffeine is one of the most "sacred cows" of our society. Almost everyone is a "user". Most people don't want to hear the truth or simply they have convinced themselves that "it's not that bad". Just ask yourself, "why is the amount of caffeine consumption listed on most medical forms you are given to fill out?" Believe me, these forms aren't a social thing. Caffeine has a direct negative relationship on all aspects of your health.

But once the truth is out there in print for those who would read it and apply these truths to their own bodily symptoms, maybe we can change some opinions as well as behavior. I love the taste of coffee and I suppose as a flavoring agent we could satisfy our taste buds, but personally I am not willing to pay the very, very high price from the side effects.

The following truths and myths are in outline form for easy reference.

Caffeine:

Raises blood pressure

Contributes to adrenal exhaustion

Increases ulcer risk

Contributes to hormone imbalance and many health disorders in women

Raises blood cholesterol levels which increases the likelihood of a STROKE

Does not provide energy – only chemical stimulation

Women and children have a limited ability to detoxify the drug (caffeine)

Increases stress level hormones that can lead to pain

Affects the aging process

Over 700 volatile substances in coffee have been identified

Causes heart palpitations, anxiety, insomnia, panic

1% caffeine is excreted in the urine, 99% must be detoxified by the liver

May take up to 7 days to detoxify the blood of heavy coffee users

Can take 3 weeks or more for the stress levels to return to normal

Caffeine soft drinks contain 45 to 72 mg per 12 oz. can

6 oz. of drip coffee = 100 mg caffeine

The "Cure" for Health Care Reform

6 oz percolated = 120 mg

6 oz European style boiled coffee packs = 160 mg

Coffee shop cups are from 14-20 oz

Coffee is more powerful on an empty stomach

80% of American adults drink 3-4 cups/day (60-150 mg per cup)

Heart disease patients are more at risk over 300 mg when arrhythmias can occur

Is in tea, cocoa, soft drinks, medications and chocolate

Has been found to impair motor steadiness (shaking limbs)

Is addictive and discontinuing it prompts withdrawal symptoms

Creates tension followed by fatigue

Affects mental clarity and emotional stability

Can take 3-12 hours for a cup to wear off (but not out of our system for 3 weeks)

Silent damage to adrenals, blood vessels, breasts, brain, GI tract, DNA, immune system and bones (crosses the blood brain barrier)

Is absorbed by every organ and tissue in the body and needs to be detoxified by the liver

Contains toxic chemicals and compounds

Hundreds of over the counter drugs contain caffeine and many of them interfere with the body's ability to detoxify caffeine while at the same time increasing the risk for liver disease cardiac arrhythmias and epilepsy

Some pharmaceutical drugs have been shown to increase blood levels of caffeine by more than 600%.

Liver disease can reduce the body's ability to detoxify caffeine significantly (2-6 days from a single cup of coffee)

Cigarette smokers who are trying to quit suffer a slowdown of their caffeine detox system

Does NOT help weight loss

Increases stress hormones including adrenaline, epinephrine and nor epinephrine which affects the brain, nervous system, heart rate, while increasing blood pressure

Impairs digestion – contributes to gas and bloating

Causes vascular resistance which raises blood pressure

Reduces metabolic efficiency which means less oxygen to your tissues and brain with less carbon dioxide and wastes being removed from your body.

Raises serum cortisol levels which relates to mind, mood and behavior (being in a cloud).

Affects personality leading to anger and frustration

Raises dopamine levels – a feeling of being "high"

Consumed by hundreds of million Americans each day

Stimulates your nervous system and adrenals to produce stress leading to adrenal exhaustion. Stress leads to disease, anxiety, depression, insomnia, ulcers, hypoglycemia, arthritis, headache, herpes, hypertension, asthma, and heart disease, and suppress immunity

Stress, caffeine and the suppressed function on the immune system can lead to autoimmune disorders such as rheumatoid arthritis, lupus and MS. Adrenal exhaustion = profound tiredness. Prolonged stress= serious and chronic illness

Lowers stress threshold where someone 'flies off the handle' very easily with anger, violence, frustration and depression. Does that sound like someone you know?

Drugs inhibit the body's ability to detoxify caffeine

Hormone and metabolic function may be irreversibly damaged after a certain period of time

Major personality changes leading to irritability, anxiety, unhappiness, defensive, low sex drive, headaches

Birth control pills decrease body's ability to detoxify caffeine

Interferes with restorative REM sleep cycle – you wake up feeling tired instead of restored. Moe than 250 mg caffeine leads to poor sleep quality

Fibromyalgia

The elderly detox caffeine more slowly

Blood sugar abnormalities

Malnutrition, increased loss of B vitamins, calcium and other minerals in urine

Panic attacks

1 cup coffee can reduce iron absorption by as much as 75%. Coffee and tea reduce effectiveness of iron supplements. 30% Americans have lower than normal iron

Reduces activity of monocytes and natural killer (NK) cells

Affects production of melatonin

Constriction of blood vessels in fingers = cold hands

CONCENTRATION BECOMES ONE DIMENSIONAL   You can't step back from what you're involved in. YOU LOSE YOUR HIGHER CENTERS OF REASON AND EVALUATION

Small annoyances can become major

Decreased ability to cope. Decreased ability to relax

Interferes with normal neuron firing in the brain

Creates background tension that reduces quality of life

Interferes with metabolism of GABA – biochemical that helps filter info and plan sensible action strategies

Increased incidence of mitro valve prolapse

Decreased blood circulation in the brain

Triggers panic attacks and increases frequency and intensity – anxiety, nervousness, fear, nausea, palpitations, restlessness

Moderate caffeine level doubles stress response and magnifies the stress

Fatigue and depression 3 hrs after caffeine withdrawal

Sleep disturbance common side effect of anti-depressants. Depression, then anti depressant, then sleep disturbance leading to depression

May aggravate PMS

Just 100 mg can cause a significant DECREASE IN RECALL AND REASONING

Affects mood and learning

250 mg caffeine produces a 30% decrease in brain blood flow

Increases blood pressure in brain, increased risk of stroke, reduces oxygen level of brain tissue

Increases stress hormones which accelerate aging leading to memory loss and disorientation, post traumatic stress disorder

500 mg caffeine injected into vein produces hallucinations, paranoia, panic, mania and depression in 1 hour. 500 mg ingested over a 12 hour period produces milder forms of the above

Dizziness

Can disturb sleep up to 8 hrs

Caffeine's side effects can lead to alcoholic consumption

The "Cure" for Health Care Reform

Hyperactivity in children

Bottle fed babies experience caffeine withdrawal

Chronic disturbed sleep leads to signs of emotional illness

Promotes rage - rage key factor in 2/3 fatal car crashes

Vascular resistance check above for this

Increases negative mod, decreases positive mood

Influences cardiovascular disease including stroke and hardening of the arteries,

Negative effect when taken with diet pills

Disturbs calcium metabolism

Elevates cholesterol in as little as 2 cups or more per day

Less than 300 mg day can cause cardiac arrhythmia

Tachycardia (rapid heart beat)

Ventricular premature beats after coffee ingestion

Coronary vasospasm (can shut off blood supply)

Correlation between caffeine and elevated dangerous blood levels of homocysteine which contributes to stroke, miscarriage, birth defects and possibly Alzheimer's disease

High homocysteine levels = 3 times the risk for cardiovascular disease. Caffeine depletes B vitamins which then raises homocysteine levels. B vitamin supplements help reverse this.

High homocysteine damages blood vessels. Diabetics usually have low homocysteine levels

Rheumatoid arthritis may have a defect in homocysteine metabolism.

Homocysteine accelerates free radical activity which damages nerve cells

50% of persons over 65 have elevated homocysteine levels

HOMOCYSTEINE ELIMINATES PROTECTIVE BENEFITS FROM HDL CHOLESTEROL. Caffeine raises homocysteine levels

Anxiety and stress increases production of epinephrine and cortisol which affects mood and behavior which creates more stress, hostility, and anger. Caffeine magnifies stress levels leading to higher stress hormone levels

Small artery spasms cuts off blood supply to heart for a short period of time

Tachycardia (rapid heart beat)

Caffeine depletes magnesium which helps cause rapid heartbeat

Caffeine increases adrenaline which accelerate4s blood clotting

1-2 CUPS OF COFFEE A DAY INCREASES RISK OF HEART ATTACK BY 40%

More than 36 oz. coffee a day results in creases heart attack risk FOR WOMEN by 250%. Less than 24 oz has 2 times the risk of heart attach for women

Caffeine interferes with all phases of the gastro-intestinal tract including microbial defenses, digestion, nutrient absorption, elimination , as well as the barrier that keeps foreign bodies out of the bloodstream. It affects vitamin and mineral absorption

Caustic acids in coffee contribute to IBS (irritable bowel syndrome) and ulcers

Some individuals are allergic to the chemicals that the coffee beans are treated with

Reduces melatonin levels, the hormone needed for sleep and enhancement of DNA synthesis. Sleep essential to repair tissue damage

Can contribute to carpal tunnel syndrome

Disrupts calcium, causing muscle tension

Significant amounts of caffeine in pain killers

Surgery patients are given a caffeine drip so they don't undergo withdrawal

Has diuretic effect with nutrients lost in urine, dehydration which accelerates aging

Impairs ability of the body to detoxify drugs, etc.

Caffeine can cause replication error of cells

Impairs immunity

Raises blood sugar limits, disrupts blood sugar regulating effects of insulin. High caffeine levels mimic type 2 diabetes

Raises fatty acid levels in the blood. Diabetics already have high fat blood levels and adding caffeine raises their risk for heart disease even more

Toxic effect on fetal development

Lowers DHEA hormones critical for function of immune, cardiovascular, reproductive and nervous systems

With birth control pills- caffeine can take 2 times as long to detox

Caffeine exacerbates symptoms of fibromyalgia, decreased circulation to the fingers

Impairs intestinal wall barrier leading to increased absorption of toxins into the body

Rats fed caffeine developed atrophy to their testicles and a low sperm count

Can aggravate gout

Increases pressure in the eyes of most people while decreasing the micro-circulation of the eye. Can make eyes very dry

Women detox caffeine much more slowly than men, even slower in the last 2 weeks of their menstrual cycle

Elevates cortisol which contributes to lost bone density

Significant association between caffeine intake and miscarriage

Women caffeine drinkers 2 times more likely to develop an ulcer

Studies from 90,000 women show a correlation between caffeine and hip fracture

Reduction in iron absorption resulting in lack of energy and concentration

Increase in menopausal symptoms, research studies show that eliminating caffeine can reduce menopausal symptoms

Can delay conception

Women who drank more than 300 mg caffeine per day had 2 times the rate of fetal loss in utero than those who drank less than 46 mg a day

Major risk in late spontaneous abortions, low birth weight,

Correlation between caffeine and fetal malformation, especially heart and brain

Newborns lack the enzyme to break down caffeine and will suffer withdrawal from a mother who has caffeine in her system

Commercially grown coffee is heavily sprayed with dangerous herbicides, pesticides, and fungicides with a high level on coffee beans as well as residues of carcinogens

Cola drinks have about 9 teaspoons of sugar while the acidity weakens tooth enamel

Attention deficit disorder (ADD) in children improved when caffeine and sugar were eliminated from their diets

Caffeine in cola drinks and chocolate have a much higher impact in children because a child's weight is much less than and an adult's weight

Throws off the ratio of calcium and phosphorus needed for building bones, increases calcium loss in urine

Decaf higher in acidity and has about 10 mg caffeine, not for people with ulcers and intestinal tract disorders

Methyline chloride used to extract caffeine from coffee beans

Decaf can affect blood sugar levels

Tea can inhibit iron absorption enough to cause anemia

Withdrawal symptoms:

Headache caused by increased blood flow circulation to the brain

Sluggish bowel elimination due to decreased intestinal muscle contractions

Induces fatigue, depression and brain fog. Body needs time to adjust to not getting its "fix"

Induces and magnifies stress when withdrawing

Hinders your ability to see the 'big picture'

Clearly there's no way around having your coffee and avoiding all the consequences. If you want to improve your health drastically, caffeine MUST be eliminated from your diet. If you persist in making excuses like "I love the taste" or "I need the social interaction", be prepared for the consequences which will most likely manifest in disease and shortened life expectancy.

You simply cannot jump off a building and expect not to fall.

There is a very tasty coffee alternative, it comes in 10 flavors and it's name is Teeccino. You will still have withdrawal, but mixing a substitute with your coffee and gradually decreasing the coffee amount could be very helpful. Organic decaf can also help.

Please see Reference Guide on where to purchase.

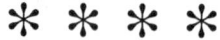

CHAPTER 7
Enzymes – The Key To Life

Enzymes are needed for every chemical action and reaction in our bodies as well as important factors in longevity, vitality, health, and weight control.

The older we become, we deplete our 'enzyme bank accounts' if we are not replacing them with raw foods and enzyme supplements. They are needed to break down every food we eat which only maintains our bodies if it is digested properly. If enough nutrients are not absorbed, the foundation is laid for a weak immune system and disease.

Merely taking vitamins does not make up for the deficiency. The supplements must be entirely natural without being refined and then have the proper enzymes for the absorption of the vitamins. Please see chapter Vitamins Anyone?

There is a belief that people with food allergies have vitamin and mineral deficiencies due to a lack of enzymes and, of course, taking the wrong supplements. Some allergies are caused by a lack of regularity in the bowel which can also be related to an enzyme deficiency.

Enzymes help to increase oxygen in the body which makes it hard for most cancers and certain anaerobic diseases (diseases that thrive in a lack of oxygen) to gain a foothold. They also can protect you from free radical damage. We need to build up our enzyme reserves for emergencies just like a 'rainy day' account.

I personally have used digestive enzymes to relieve and eliminate heartburn, intestinal gas and for WEIGHT LOSS. These enzymes can dissolve excess cholesterol in the liver and other body parts that help protect the heart while eliminating excess stored body fats that our body does not need.

The two basic classes of enzymes are metabolic and digestive. The metabolic enzymes are responsible for the overall maintenance of the body and all its systems. The digestive enzymes break down all our food through digestion which then goes on to provide the fuel. Digestive enzymes have three functions: digesting protein (proteases), carbohydrates (amylases) and fats (lipases). If we keep our enzyme levels high by taking enzyme supplements, we save our metabolic enzymes the work load of replacing them in the body and allow them to do the job they were intended to do, maintaining our basic health. 50% of our daily protein goes to enzyme production.

Eating raw food means that the food has not been heated about 145 degrees (F.), the temperature that enzymes cannot survive.

Supplementing digestive enzymes with our food literally saves our enzyme storage bank and allows our bodies to conserve metabolic enzymes for our much needed bodily maintenance. As with almost everything else, enzyme production decreases with age.

Enzyme deficiency is reported to speed up the development of diseases such as cancer, arthritis, aging, heart and organ problems, etc. Impure water, air pollution, smoking, and improper food all are contributors.

As stated earlier, heat destroys enzymes. If the food is hot to the touch, the enzymes are gone. By contrast, animals in the wild that are eating properly are usually very healthy.

Athletic activity uses up more enzymes than normal so it is wise to supplement with enzymes after exercising of any kind.

One of the first organs affected by an enzyme deficiency is the pancreas. As our food becomes more deficient in enzymes, the pancreas must borrow enzyme substances from other parts of the body to function. This causes one's pancreas to overwork and thus become enlarged. Depending on how long this abuse continues, the way is paved for pancreatic cancer.

If enzymes are not being replaced from supplements or raw foods, one can readily see how the incidence of diabetes is on the rise. I know this sounds like an oversimplification, but it really makes perfect sense, an overworked pancreas will fail. One may argue that heredity plays a major role, but consider the fact that families usually have the same diets. This can contribute to a shortened life span by accelerating the aging process.

The pancreas is the largest organ producing digestive enzymes. Enzymes also aid in the conversion of food into muscle, bone, nerves and glands while helping to store excess food for energy and rebuilding the body. The most potent digestive enzymes are amylase and protease.

It is believed that human breast milk has extra lipase enzymes to compensate for a deficiency in the pancreatic juice of the human infant, therefore if one is bottle feeding, a lipase enzyme added to the formula could go a long way to preventing baby's indigestion. Breast milk has all the necessary enzymes and is considered a raw food while bottle formula has no enzymes.

The continual depletion and absence of enzymes at mealtime is thought to be a major contributor in the formation of disease and malfunction of the human body and frankly, I agree. A complete digestive enzyme at mealtime can virtually abolish heartburn, unless you have some other underlying cause for the heartburn.

While heating food destroys all enzymes, frying goes a step further. The extra high heat actually damages protein and forms new chemical components in the process, Baking, however, employs a dry heat so the destruction of all of the enzymes is the same as boiling.

Canned food simply is the worst (other than frying). The canning process not only destroys all the enzymes, but the majority of vitamins as well. One is simply left with calories.

Let's examine what percentage of raw food we are ingesting. While eating 75% raw foods is ideal, most of us are consuming only 10-15% raw foods (with enzymes), if that. While writing this chapter I'm trying to increase my raw foods, but it's difficult. Ingesting certain raw foods can lead to parasites and a possible bacterial invasion. Try supplementing with a digestive enzyme at each meal, preferably just after a heavy protein meal so that the enzyme does not have to compete with the digestive stomach acids and will help compensate for the lack of raw food. Mega Food has a good digestive enzyme called "Megazymes" or Progressive Labs "Digestin".

Here's an interesting factor. Continued use of refined sugars and carbohydrates, in addition to leading to obesity, has a deleterious effect on our pituitary, thyroid and pancreas glands. In short, poor nutrition destroys the proper functioning of our organs.

Decreased enzymes in the body leads to an enlarged pancreas which, in turn, causes it to waste more enzymes than a smaller pancreas. The pancreas will steal from metabolic enzymes (those enzymes involved in the body's metabolism) and convert them to digestive enzymes. This deprives the rest of the body of some necessary metabolic enzymes needed for the body to run properly and causes your brain, organs arteries and tissues to suffer from an enzyme shortage. An enlarged pancreas will waste up to 3 times as many enzymes, thus continuing a vicious downward spiral toward malfunction.

Refined white sugar throws the body out of balance because when searching for vitamins, minerals, and enzymes, it recognizes the deficiency and signals the appetite center of the brain to call for more food. This causes chronic over stimulation of the pancreas and pituitary glands.

Refined sugar also leads to increased cholesterol levels. In laboratory animals sugar was found to increase the incidence of kidney disease. Consider the high incidence of kidney disease in our pets. Most of our cat and dog food has sugar and absolutely no enzymes because it is heated. Just ask any vet how many incidences of kidney disease they encounter. It is much, much higher than it should be. I have always been very careful to see to it that there are no drugs, antibiotics, hormones and sugar in my pet's food. We need to factor in the high cost of vet bills which makes the higher quality food less expensive than the cheap food.

Foods that have been irradiated by microwaves, even raw foods, have had all their enzymes destroyed. By ingesting this type of food, one could seriously question what type of genetic mutations this could lead to in the human body.

Enteric coated enzyme tablets are designed to by pass the gastric juices of the stomach and dissolve in the intestine which is very effective for relieving inflammation in the body such as arthritis,

They can also assist a malfunctioning pancreas.

Some additional facts about enzymes:

Enzymes can reduce cholesterol, regulate insulin levels, normalize weight and help with skin conditions.

Lipase is useful for psoriasis and fat metabolism.

Undigested or the wrong food can detrimentally change tissues and organs.

Most persons over the age of 50 have an abnormal pituitary gland caused by heat treated, refined, enzyme free food. Cooked food over stimulates the endocrine system

The major portion of digestive enzymes is used for protein.

Fasting allows body to heal and recover digestive enzymes.

Rheumatoid arthritis, as well as other forms of arthritis, may be an enzyme deficiency disease from an inability to deal adequately with protein digestion and metabolism.

There is laboratory proof that cancer patients have disturbed enzyme chemistry.

There is a correlation between allergies and low enzymes in body from incompletely digested protein molecules.

Cardiovascular disease can result from incomplete metabolism of fats and low lipase activity.

Enzymes weaken with age.

A shortage of enzymes can cause cholesterol deposits in arterial walls. Clogged arteries can lead to heart attack, high blood pressure, and/or a stroke.

Discordant sound (awful music or loud obnoxious noise) can disrupt enzymes.

THE BOTTOM LINE HERE IS IF WE SUPPLEMENT PROPER EATING WITH ENZYMES, WE CAN GO A LONG WAY TOWARD ELIMINATING ILLNESS AND DISEASE AND THEREFORE BE LESS DEPENDENT ON OUR HEALTH INSURANCE.

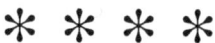

CHAPTER 8
Water

I hear it all the time. "My water is just fine, I have one of those filters on my faucet". This is like putting a band aid on an incision that is the result of major surgery. It simply is not true that this carbon filter is eliminating all the poisons in your water. The charcoal filter will take the chorine out of the water and make it taste better, but only for a short while. After a short while the bacteria build up in the filter will leach out of the filter into your drinking water. Yuk!

Chorine in the shower can strip protein from hair and skin, irritate eyes and cause dandruff.

It has been recently discovered that there are drugs not only in our drinking water, but drugs were also found in the top 10 bottled water brands. (Eyewitness News October 15, 2008, Charles Gibson).

What to do? People and pets are not immune to this type of poisoning. We do not have any special filters in our bodies other than the normal organs, e.g. liver, kidneys, etc. which have to overwork to try to get rid of these chemicals, Some of these chemicals end up being stored in the body.

The drugs in the water drugs can also desensitize us to drugs we may need in the future. This simply means that the body has reached its tolerance level from ingesting the drug, and it will not work when prescribed by your doctor.

The answer is distilled water which should only be purchased in a glass bottle because the nature of this water is osmotic (it draws out non organic substances). This is wonderful in the body but it leaches the plastic from the plastic bottle into the distilled water. This is okay for your iron but not for drinking. Today's home distillers have either a stainless steel storage tank or a polycarbonate bottle for storage. Polycarbonate is actually a very stable type of thick plastic that can contain the distilled water without leaching the plastic into the water.

The EPA standards of acceptable pollutants in today's water does not take into account the cumulative effect of these toxins being stored in our bodies as well as that of our pets. The last count I know of was 75,000 chemical compounds in our water. Many countries have banned the use of fluoride (rat poison) in their drinking water We have not banned fluoride in out water and yet we have one of the highest rates of tooth decay in the world The Physicians Desk Reference actually shows mottling of the teeth and heart problems as just a couple of the side effects of fluoride. The National Cancer Institute has linked 50,000 cancer deaths a year in humans to fluoride. Our pets are not immune to this either.

Our tap drinking water also contains heavy metals such as lead, arsenic, aluminum, nitrates, iron, radioactivity, radon, mercury etc.

Many people think that their wells are safe. Wells can contain runoff from acid rain, pesticides, fertilizer, as well as a list too long to mention here.

According to the International Bottled Water Association, there is a 1 in 4 chance that your bottled water has been drawn from municipal taps which means they are contaminated with the above toxins. These are major name brands we have always taken for granted as being pure.

Bottled water info – most plastic bottle containers for water leach plastic right into the water.

Bottled water still has varying amount of nitrates, fluoride, aluminum, lead, arsenic, mercury, etc. etc.

I have used a home distiller for over 25 years and have been very satisfied. These distillers remove over 99% of chemicals and toxins. I know of no other process that works as well. Again, please see the following chart.

Some advantages of home distillation is that the units effectively remove bacteria, viruses, fluoride, nitrates, heavy metals, asbestos and all minerals.

There is a standing controversy that distilled water leaches minerals from our bodies. The true fact is that it only leaches inorganic minerals and substances from the body, leaving the "good stuff" alone. However, it is these inorganic minerals that cause the body to stiffen with age. Drinking distilled water actually helps break up these hardened deposits around the joints. It also helps prevent these inorganic substances from hanging out in the body's organs and causing disease.

Someone recently told me that I would be experiencing a loss of mobility in the not too distant future as a consequence of aging. I replied that inasmuch as I have been drinking distilled water for many years this wasn't going to be a problem.

Water, in itself, contains very little organic minerals only inorganic. A high quality diet along with the right supplements should provide us with all the minerals we need.

Regarding the cost, home distillers range from the low $300's to a couple of thousand dollars for a large stainless steel unit with all the bells and whistles. Compare the cost to operate (about 25-35 cents per gallon depending upon your electric bill rate) to the price of a gallon of store bought bottled water. Usually the more expensive the unit, the faster it will distill. The larger units give off a considerable amount of heat but have a pumping system that enables you to keep the distiller in the basement and pump on demand to a special kitchen sink faucet. I particularly like not having to transport bottle after bottle from the grocery store.

DEPENDING ON YOUR USE A HOME UNIT CAN PAY FOR ITSELF IN UNDER A YEAR WHILE LASTING FOR MANY, MANY YEARS (stainless steel units can last for 20 years, and then longer after being refurbished). Waterwise and Pure and Secure and two reliable companies I know of. Please see Reference Guide for Pure and Secure's substantial discounts to readers of this book.

The following chart at the end of this chapter shows just what today's filter systems DON'T DO!

Comparison of Water Treatment Technologies

	Sediment Filter	Carbon Filter	Deionization	Reverse Osmosis	Steam Distillation
Arsenic	○	○	●	◑	●
Bacteria	○	○	○	◑	●
Cadmium	○	○	●	●	●
Calcium	○	○	●	●	●
Chlorides	○	○	●	●	●
Chlorine	○	●	○	●¹	●¹
Cryptosporidium	○	○	○	●	●
Detergents	○	◑	●	●	●
Fluorides	○	○	●	●	●
Lead	○	○	●	●	●
Magnesium	○	○	●	●	●
Nitrate	○	○	◑	◑	●
Organics ·	○	●	○	●¹	●¹
Pesticides	○	●	○	●¹	●¹
Phosphates	○	○	●	●	●
Radon	○	○	●	●	●
Sediment	●	◑	●	●	●
Sodium	○	○	●	●	●
Sulfates	○	◑	●	●	●
Viruses	○	○	○	○	●

○ Ineffective or No Reduction   ◑ Significant Reduction   ● Complete or Significant Reduction

¹ Plus Carbon Filtration

CHAPTER 9
We Need Warning Labels
On Our Foods

This has been done for cigarettes and tobacco products and was a long time coming, now the public needs to warned on other hidden dangers and then come to an informed decision. Here are some suggestions:

"WARNING: This product contains nitrates and nitrites, known carcinogens (cancer causing agents) and can be harmful to your health"

For example, if some bacon and ham manufacturers do not have these harmful substances in their product, why do the others?

"WARNING: This produce has been grown out of the country and has been sprayed with an undetermined amount of pesticides, a certain percentage of which you will ingest"

"WARNING: This product contains 75% or more fillers and is an incomplete food source"

"WARNING: This product contains a high level of refined sugars which have been know to be a precursor to diabetes"

"WARNING: This product contains carcinogens which have been linked to cancer"

"WARNING: This beauty product contains SLS which has been linked to causing changes in hormone levels, eye irritation, gender confusion and cancer"

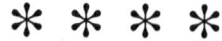

CHAPTER 10
Explicit Dangers Of Microwaves

I can hear it now, "microwaves are perfectly safe, I've been using mine for years and nothing bad has happened". Well, nothing bad that you know of, but let's consider the scientific facts. Stay in denial if you choose, but those of you who want the truth, read on.

Microwaves change the molecular content of foods. This is especially dangerous for baby formula. The baby formulas on the market have fewer nutrients than breast milk and to microwave these formulas really adds insult to injury because it severely depletes any nutrients.

It has been documented that when a nurse heated blood with a micro-wave and when she gave it to a patient in a transfusion, the patient DIED FROM THE TRANSFUSION. The microwaving of the blood changed its molecular structure to the extent that it was toxic to the patient. Imagine what microwaving does to the food we eat.

Studies have also shown that blood drawn from persons eating microwaved food had lower hemoglobin levels, lower white blood cell counts (our immune fighters) HIGHER CHOLESTEROL LEVELS, and brainwave disturbances leading to memory loss and sleep disorders. This is no bargain to save a few minutes of time.

Microwaving interferes with the natural process of the body's cellular repair as the food molecules are torn apart in the process of heating in the microwave and are not put back in their original state. This also reduces the body's oxygen content by producing hydrogen peroxide and carbon monoxide in the body.

Studies have also shown that microwaving produces carcinogens, even when thawing foods. Lymphatic disorders were observed leading to decreased ability to prevent cancers with an increased rate of cancer cell formation in the blood. Also, there has been shown to be a 60-90% decreased food value with a loss of vitamins as well such as vitamin E, C, essential minerals, etc.

In researching this subject, I have come across some information that was completely new to me. It's called "microwave sickness" and comes from eating microwaved food. It is characterized by low blood pressure, slow pulse, can include headache, dizziness, eye pain, insomnia, stomach pain, nervous tension, inability to concentrate, hair loss, plus an increased incidence of appendicitis, cataracts, reproductive problems and inability to prevent certain types of cancers. Of equal importance are higher levels of brainwave disturbance causing loss of memory, loss of ability to concentrate, and interrupted sleep patterns.

You may be thinking, "well, if using a microwave oven is so harmful, how come almost everyone has and uses them?" There are many answers to this. First of all, there has been a massive 'brainwashing' of the

American public that the microwave is a blessing, a real time saver. Those magic words "time saver" is all most overworked people have to hear.

Second, most people are not scientists and can't conceptualize how this can be harmful. This is more than a smoking gun, I invite you to investigate further. The web is a good place to begin, you'll see I'm not making this up.

Third, since microwaving is very subtle and one cannot see the damage it is doing. It's hard to connect the dots when your body starts to malfunction – you blame something else.

Finally, as a scientist, I have personally NEVER used a microwave oven simply because it makes no sense to injure myself. And when I'm out of my home and stop for something to eat, I request that the cooks do not "nuke" my food.

The bottom line is the time you save isn't worth the major damage to your body you incur. Remember, everything negative you remove from your life has a positive impact on your body.

Please see chapter on Harmful EMF Fields

* * * *

CHAPTER 11
Joan's Picks

The following foods I consider to be way ahead of their time and it is my hope that by popular demand more manufacturers will follow their example.

BREAKFAST

Organic eggs (free of hormones and antibiotics) These are much better for you than the fake ones because they are fake food.

Applegate Farms Hickory Smoked Turkey Bacon

Nature's Path assorted cereals, Barbara's Shredded Oats

Kashi assorted cereals, Island Vanilla Shredded Wheat, your kids will eat it

Organic fruit when possible, otherwise conventional fruit

Organic unsweetened fruit juices

Ezekial assorted breads and English muffins, made from sprouted grains and much better for the body than regular whole grain breads

Food For Life assorted breads, English muffins also made from sprouted grains

Organic jams jellies sweetened with fruit juice or just completely natural

Organic unsalted butter, you don't need any extra salt in your butter, there's enough salt in most other foods. Most margarine is simply heated oil and, in my opinion, has a negative health benefit.

Raw honey

LUNCH

Organic cheeses, must be "organic" as there will be no antibiotics and hormones in the milk. Cheeses made from heated oil belongs in the garbage, not the refrigerator

Cold cuts whose label states "No antibiotics, nitrates, or nitrites (Applegate Farms)

Whole grain or sprouted grain breads (must be 100% whole grains)

Health soups in the can or a health food frozen dinner – works in a "pinch" but read the labels carefully for serving sizes and salt (sodium) 2 serving sizes = double the salt. Amy's, Health Valley Organic, Imagine Organic (canned variety) have some very tasty ones.

Leftovers from your healthy dinner last night. Always good to make extra and have the leftovers for lunch

Organic yoghurt sweetened with cane juice not sugar. There is a difference in the manufacturing process. Stonyfield Farms is one manufacaturer.

Vegetarian chicken deluxe sandwich by Sunneen Health Foods

DINNER

Rancher ground turkey for meat loafs, burgers, meatballs, etc.\

Rancher hot dogs, beef ,chicken, turkey

Free range organic chicken, whole, cut up, wings

Organic steak, ground beef

Turkey sausage cooked in tomato sauce over brown rice pasta

Organic lamb cubes for stew or as a roast

Organic veal cubes for stew or shish kabob

Wild caught fresh fish (shellfish should be at a minimum)

SNACKS

Finn Crisp plus 5 whole grains thin crisp bread crackers

Susie's Italian Herbs Spelt crackers, other flavors available but check for the whole grain flavors

Pop Chips original flavor has no sugar, these chips are popped like pop corn

SWEETS

Organicville ice cream

Back to Nature cookies – cranberry pecan granola

Grade B maple syrup which has all the minerals left in

Manna Organic Fruit and Nut Bread

Raw honey

PERSONAL PRODUCTS

Crystal roll on body deodorant (no aluminum, very effective) Also comes in Lightly Scented, spray and stick in Lavender & White Tea, Pomegranate, Chamomile & Green Tea, as well as Unscented.

Zia Ultilmate Oil Free Moisture (moisturizer for face, I love this), expensive but can last a while.

Abra lotions, creams, body scrubs, therapy and detox baths, etc. Outstanding line of products made with dispersing organic extracts, volcanic minerals and rich essential oils.

Sensodyne Pronamel toothpaste – while this product contains some sodium fluoride it is very effective in helping to hardening tooth enamel.

HOUSEHOLD PRODUCTS

BioKleen Line of kitchen, bathroom, and laundry cleaners. These are excellent www.biokleenhome.com

7th Generation Household Cleaners,

Mister Max Anti-Icky-Poo Unscented Pet Urine and Odor Eliminator
Non-Scents Multi-Strain Bacterial Solution
They have other formulas but this is the one I prefer.
www.mistermax.com

VITAMINS

Whey protein powder for building muscle

MegaFood whole food vitamin line

Glandulars from Nutricology

Progressive Labs
www.progressivelabs.com
20% discount with mention of this book
1-800-527-9512

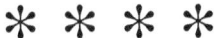

ALTERNATIVE HEALTH REMEDIES

CHAPTER 12
Ailments And Diseases

This chapter will attempt to guide you into more favorable treatments for the following illnesses and diseases. This is not intended to be a substitute for a doctor's advice nor does it recommend abandoning life support medication such as immune depressant drugs needed to avoid the body rejecting a transplant.

Please see Reference Guide for more complete information.

ACCELERATED AGING – due to impurities in the food, water, air, and excess stress. High quality food based natural supplements facilitate longer telomeres, a substance that keeps your chromosomes from unraveling when body cells divide. These telomeres get shorter as we age and keeping them from shortening through natural supplements helps keep them longer while keeping us younger. Omega 3 fatty acids (krill oil) have been reported to help keep those "tellys" longer.

ALCOHOLISM – It is reported that more than 70% of alcoholics are in denial, thinking that they don't have a problem. Alcohol kills off brain cells. Treatment usually requires some form of therapy, natural diet, The herb kudzu is reported to help with cravings, milk thistle and dandelion to help restore liver function, and St. John's Wort for depression.

ALLERGIES – Now that the climate is getting warmer, the allergy (pollen) season is extending. Have you ever heard an advertisement aimed at stopping allergies in the first place? The only advertisements I see and hear are those designed to suppress allergy symptoms by taking all that medication, however, this comes at a price. By clogging your liver with medication you simply make yourself more vulnerable to increased symptoms.

The proactive approach is best. Imagine pollen season comes and the only way you will notice this season is by seeing pollen on the trees or on the ground.

THESE ALLERGIES ARE NOT NORMAL!! Your body is telling you that you are out of balance. Eating a more balanced healthy diet along with some colon cleansing should go a long way toward eliminating your allergies. Another factor is obesity. The more overweight you are the more likely you are to suffer from allergies along with a long list of other maladies. Not to worry, there is a chapter on Weight Loss.

Now if you have a sensitivity to a particular food or foods, it's best to avoid these foods. I have an allergy to chocolate (just terrible) and ever once in a while I succumb. When I was younger, I used to get a few hives, but now I find my immune system is weakened by it and I usually contract a cold. A chocolate craving can be the result of a magnesium deficiency. MegaFood magnesium is the vitamin of choice I use should I find the craving very strong.

Now, not to rub it in, but my theory works. Here it is pollen allergy season again and the only way I found out was that it was on the news.

ALZHEIMERS -This dreaded 'time bomb' disease that arrives usually later in life may not be as mysterious as one might imagine. The brain shrinks and there is loss of some of one's nervous system. Once again, I believe prevention is the key.

Signs of this disease include sleep disturbances, physical or verbal out-bursts. emotional distress, restlessness, delusions and/or hallucinations.

Alzheimers is the result of sticky plaque build up in the brain, this defini-tion being oversimplified. It is reported that 10% of the population is expe-riencing Alzheimers by the age of 65 and 50% by the age of 80.

Studies have shown a connection between Alzheimers and aluminum from the brain tissue of deceased patients. This is not as confusing as it sounds. We certainly don't go down to an aluminum manufacturing plant and have lunch, however, an awareness of which foods aluminum is present and by simply avoiding those foods altogether could ultimately prevent this disease.

Aluminum is present in aluminum cans, porcelain crowns, antacids, tap water, baked goods, regular tea, beer, toothpaste, deodorants, cosmetics and what I consider to be most deadly, is the use of aluminum cookware including those 'non stick' pans which give off an array of chemicals while cooking. Aluminum foil is probably safe if it does not come in contact with the food and is used to simply catch spilled food. THERE ARE FOODS, DEODORANTS, COSMETICS, STAINLESS STEEL COOKWARE AVAILABALE, ALL WILTHOUT ALUMINUM. YOU SIMPLY MUST READ THE LABELS.

Alzheimers patients can benefit from a natural diet, sunlight, extra sleep, MegaFood B and C vitamins, Vitamin E (complete), ginko, and antioxidants.

Important to note here that countries that use the spice tumeric on a regular basis have remarkably low incidences of Alzheimers. Also, glutathione helps remove or neutralize dangerous substances in the body including toxic metals.

ARTHRITIS/JOINT INFLAMMATION - Rheumatoid arthritis is an auto-immune disease where the body confuses healthy tissue for foreign invaders and the body attacks the healthy tissue.

This type of arthritis not only attacks the joints, but other organs as well. Some natural remedies that may prove helpful would be Thymus glandular which can improve the immune system as well as vitamins A, D, and C. Osteoarthritis attacks the joints and bone. A remedy I have found very helpful is Collagen JS (chicken cartilage which provides collagen) and Glucosomine Chrondroitin by Pure Encapsulations.

Connective tissue aches and pains have a variety of causes which include:

Nutritional deficiencies

Repeated trauma to cartilage and the connective tissue that holds joints together

Repeated strain causing microscopic tears in connective tissue around joints and tendon sheaths, e.g. carpal tunnel syndrome

Inflammatory reactions to these connective tissue strains due to a prosta-glandin imbalance secondary to dietary choices (such as too much meat and milk and not enough foods with omega-3 & 6 fatty acids

Lack of the body's cortisone responses to check the inflammation

Enzyme replacement therapy can be very helpful as well as progesterone cream. Please see chapter on Enzymes and For Women Only.

ASTHMA - When I was 25 years old and in excellent health, I was pregnant with my first child. Five months into the pregnancy I developed a severe problem with my breathing. My doctor's diagnosis was "pregnancy induced asthma" and prescribed a drug which put me in 'outer space'. I knew there must be another way and fortunately the answer came quickly.

I had just refilled my prenatal vitamins at the drug store and upon arriving home, the prescription label fell off revealing the actual potency of the vitamins. To my surprise, not only were the vitamin potencies less than my regular vitamins, but there was absolutely no vitamin E in the formula.

I immediately started back on my regular vitamins (that had the vitamin E included) and my asthma cleared up the same day .I have since discovered that vitamin E is best taken in its total complete form: d-alpha-tocopherol, d-beta-tocopherol, d-gamma-tocopherol, d-delta-tocopherol as well as the alpha, beta, gamma, delta tocotrienols.

If the vitamin E prefix reads "dl" instead of "d" on the label, this indicates that the vitamin E is a synthetic and not the natural product.

I recently spoke to a young mother who was taking at least one immune depressing drug for asthma. She knew of the side effects but seemed unwilling to try anything natural to help her breathe. Interestingly, while I was in her kitchen her husband whipped out one of the name brand toxic cleaners and starting wiping down the kitchen countertops. I don't have asthma, but the smell of the chemicals in this cleaner was giving ME trouble breathing.

My comments and suggestions for her to rid herself of the asthma and medication fell on deaf ears because she needed the approval of her doctor who I'm reasonably sure has no idea of how full spectrum vitamin E can help abolish asthma..

Have you ever wondered why so many seniors have breathing issues, and are on oxygen with various forms of medication for breathing? Part of the reason for this is that we start to lose lung tissue each year starting around age 40-45. This directly affects one's ability to breathe. Combined with allergic reactions to improper food, air pollution (both indoor and outdoor) and we have a recipe for labored breathing and lung disorders.

A helpful solution is Clear Lungs by Ridgecrest Herbals (Red Label, the Blue label is homeopathic, but I prefer the herbal). Cardio exercise will help strengthen your heart and lungs and is recommended unless you have some medical condition that would prevent you from doing so.

NOTE: If you breathing problem is very severe, you probably will have to continue on your medication, however, you may be able to lessen the amount of medication you take and possibly wean off it entirely. YOU SHOULD HAVE THE COUNSEL OF A DOCTOR WHO IS SCHOOLED IN NATURAL MEDICINE to accomplish this.

The side effects of these natural products are increased ability to breathe without pain vs. potentially some very nasty, horrible side effects of the medication(s) such as a lung infection. If you develop a lung infection, your breathing could very well be worse than before you took the medication.

ATHEROSCLEROSIS – Niacin probably produces the greatest increase in high density lipoproteins (HDL) levels. (HDL's help remove plaque from artery walls). Recommended is the no-flush type. In addition, the polyphenols from pomegranate supplements decreased carotid artery thickness by 13% after 3 months and 35% after 12 months.. Also, please see cholesterol.

AUTISM – is thought to be caused by diminished oxygen in the brain and/or immunological mediated inflammatory condition in the gut. 1 in 6 children have autism says the latest statistic. There are reportedly stem cell treatments underway for this affliction.

AUTOIMMUNE DISEASE – there is a list of 63 autoimmune disorders on the internet, rheumatoid arthritis, fibromyalgia, MS, and lupus to name a few.

Let's examine just what autoimmune disease really is. It is one's own immune system gone into overdrive, hyperactive for the record. Basically, it's an immune system that is malfunctioning below normal limits. The autoimmune immune system turns and attacks one's own body. Because a lowered immune function simply does not do the job it was intended to do, namely ward off infections and disease, our bodies are severely compromised.

Now the standard medical treatment for autoimmune disease is to prescribe drugs that depress one's immune system to counteract the overdrive. Those nasty side effects you hear about are really true, heart failure, cancer, death, (also called a "fatal event") etc.

IT'S LIKE TAKING AN AIDS PILL. Persons with AIDS are trying desperately to increase their lowered immune response and here you have persons actually taking medication to depress their immune system which invites all types of infection and disease. WHAT'S WRONG WITH THIS BACKWARDS PICTURE?

Here's what is wrong. A hyperactive immune system which can be responsible for autoimmune disease is a system that is malfunctioning only in the other direction. The causes of the malfunction need to be eliminated and some natural immune boosters need to be given.

One of the main causes of anything malfunctioning in our bodies is chemicals and drugs in our systems. We ingest so many chemicals from our food and the air we breathe on a daily basis that the cumulative effect is staggering over a period of time. Our bodies simply were not made to cope with all these foreign invaders.

To add insult to injury, drugs are prescribed for many diseases and give symptomatic relief for a while, but ultimately can do more harm that good.

Please, read the labels on your food. If you can't pronounce it, there's a high probability it's a "no no". Even some of the added vitamins can be synthetic. One of my favorite examples is bread which should contain about 5 basic ingredients, whole grain flour, water, egg, yeast, salt.

Some natural whole grain breads contain a variety of nuts and seeds added to the basic ingredients, such as French Meadow Hemp Bread which, by the way, has 13 grams of protein per 2 slices.

Count the number of ingredients in the loaf of bread you've been buying. The ones I have seen in the stores must have 35, 40, or more ingredients. Would it surprise you if you were to learn that most of these ingredients were toxic fillers? Now multiply this by a whole list of other toxic ingredients in your other food. Who has a chance to be healthy?

The goal is not to live this way, paying no attention to what we are eating and breathing because we have health insurance when (not if) we get sick.

We should rarely if ever, need our health insurance. If the majority of people did this, our rates would be very low. The more demand we put on our health care system the more rates will go up and services will go down.

Is anyone listening?

BLOOD PRESSURE – one of the chief causes of high blood pressure is the narrowing of the arteries due to plaque build up. This constriction causes the heart to work harder as it struggles to oxygenate the body using more force. A helpful partial solution is to clear out the plaque using a natokinase enzyme with an enteric coating.

Pomegranate has shown to cause a drop in systolic blood pressure by 21% in a 12 month period.

It goes without saying to refrain from fatty foods and trans fats. A no flush niacin works to increase HDL and lower cholesterol and thus help remove the plaque as higher LDL cholesterol can be associated with restricted blood vessels.

The nattokinase enzyme will have a slight blood thinning effect, therefore, if you are taking blood thinning medication, you may have to have your doctor adjust your medication. A doctor who is not into natural healing may not know how to do this and most likely will not recommend this type of treatment.

CANCER - It is this author's strong opinion that most, if not all cancer is preventable. The same scenario plays over and over again. At some point in time, from infancy to older adulthood, a person isn't feeling well and visits the doctor for a diagnosis. Through various tests the cancer is discovered from a melanoma (skin cancer) to advanced widespread organ or bone cancer throughout the body which most of the time is quite fatal. I believe most people believe that this is the luck of the draw or a cancer gene that has just activated.

Let's go back in time for a different and more plausible answer. Cancer, for the most part, is less complex than we are led to believe. It is an imbalance of the human body's tissues and when the imbalance in the body is in the correct proportions, the cancer begins to grow. Cancer, by definition is simply human cells gone haywire and growing in places that compromise and kill the body's normal functioning cells (malignant hyperplasia). The answer lies in learning what causes this imbalance and preventing it in the first place.

First of all, there is improper nutrition which consists of food with chemicals and all kinds of processing, additives, dyes, carcinogens, refining, etc. We assume that most food sold at the supermarkets is fit to eat, but in reality if we look closely at the labels of all the food we are eating, we discover we are literally eating pounds and pounds of chemicals, additives each year from hormones added to the feed of the animals that supply our meat and poultry, chemical sprays on the produce.

Second, impure water. Please see Chapter on Water.

Third, air pollution which replaces some of the oxygen in our tissues for chemicals. This is a perfect environment for cancer to proliferate (grow)

Fourth, an enzyme deficiency which allows the cells to become imbalanced. There is a chapter devoted to enzymes which goes into great detail.

Fifth, a progesterone imbalance. Cancers of female organs can be from an estrogen dominant, low progesterone imbalance. The hormone progesterone decreases the cell proliferation rate (growing). It helps fibroid tissue, endometriosis, and fibrocystic breast tissue return back to their normal state.

There is a saliva test for progesterone levels. It is only measured in saliva because of the size of the molecules, a blood test will not be accurate.

If we are follow the above physiological rules, the odds of a person contracting cancer should be greatly reduced.

CHOLESTEROL – The most common for of treatment for high cholesterol is the administration of statin drugs. These statins help to shut down production of cholesterol in the liver which in essence interferes with the liver's normal functioning. Other drugs block absorption in the intestines. In addition, these drugs block the production of CoQ10 which is necessary for heart muscle to function properly. One of the main side effects of statin drugs is heart failure (what a surprise). Statins also lead to muscle tissue breakdown which also affects the muscle tissue of the heart and it has been reported that one of the adverse side effects of statin drugs is it contributes to the sticky plaque in the brain linked to Alzheimers.

Recent research shows that women should have an HDL reading above 50 while men should have an HDL reading above 40.

Conversely, a no-flush niacin supplement significantly lowers the LDL (bad) cholesterol by increasing the HDL (good) cholesterol. The HDL is responsible for helping remove the plaque from the arterial walls as well preventing it from forming in the first place.

Nattokinase is an enzyme that helps remove the plaque from the walls of blood vessels and arteries. It should be taken an empty stomach with no food taken for 45 minutes. SOME MANUFACTURERS DO NOT SPECIFY THIS ON THEIR INSTRUCTIONS AND IF TAKEN WITH FOOD, THE ENZYME WILL BE DESTROYED.

Other helpful supplements are red yeast rice, guggul lipids for reducing platelet stickiness and beta glucan and especially the enzyme, nattokinase. This enzyme needs to be purchased with an enteric coating as the ones on the market without this coating will be considerably weakened by stomach acid if not completely destroyed.

COMMON COLD OR VIRUS – Oil Of Oregano by North American Herb and Spice, gel caps are recommended as the liquid has to be very diluted.

CONSTIPATION- food grade diatomaceous earth, cleans out the bowel, rids one of parasites. The chief causes of constipation are white refined sugar and white flour which have no fiber and clog up the intestines. Herbal cleansers and increasing fiber in your diet also works very well. You can also change your breakfast cereal to Nature's Path Organic Smart Bran which has psyllium added to the bran.

DEPRESSION- baring a personal tragedy of some sort, here are some more simple causes of depression:

A misalignment of the first cervical neck vertebrae (Atlas) can cause depression and is easily corrected by a chiropractic adjustment.

The time of the year during the winter solstice of December 20 through March 20 when the days are the shortest and offer the least sunlight into the eye can give rise to depression (SAD disorder). Full spectrum lighting, both fluorescent and incandescent, can give some relief.

Anti-depressant drugs can have the side effect of depression. A food based B vitamin complex such as MegaFood can help. Likewise, Omega 3 and St. John's Wort supplements.

Refusing to eliminate a person from your life who just plain depresses you.

DIABETES- from the 2011 national diabetes fact sheet 25.8 million children and adults have diabetes, (11% 20 years or older, 27% of population past 65 years old) prediabetic 79 million. It has been linked to heart disease, high blood pressure, blindness, kidney disorders, nervous system disorders, amputations, with a 2-4 times higher incidence of death.

Diabetes 2, the most common form of diabetes, results from the pancreas parts wearing out. This is caused to a large degree by refined sugar which causes one's pancreas to go into overdrive on a daily basis. This is something you don't really see or feel until it's too late and you require medication or insulin.

Depending on how severe your condition is, a pancreas glandular can offer some much needed support to an ailing pancreas. Needless to say, all refined sugar and white flour products should be avoided. Please see chapters on Glandulars, Sugar, Sugar Everywhere and The Hidden Dangers of White Flour.

Refined sugar is in almost every food imaginable, bread, frozen dinners, foods that are not intended to be sweet to the point where the average American consumes an unbelievable amount of sugar each year.

Declare war, read the labels. Every ingredient that ends in "ose" or "ol" is a sugar, such as fructose, sorbitol. It can be done. You can buy products that don't have added sweeteners, but initially it will take a little time to discover them.

The best place is the health food store. They have cereals, ketchup, breads, etc. without sugar or with a natural unrefined sweetener, but you still have to read the labels. Another key word is "unrefined cane sugar". Simply stating "cane sugar" usually means it's refined.

One of my pet peeves in the world of subterfuge is "brown sugar". Brown sugar is refined white sugar with molasses added. Not natural at all.

Stevia is a natural sweetener from a plant you can purchase at the health food store and use for baking and sweetening at home. Some of those "other" no calorie sweeteners have been proven to be carcinogenic.

Now it's time to support your body's own pancreas with digestive enzymes in addition to a pancreas glandular. It is important to take a digestive enzyme with each meal or heavy snack. The pancreas glandular is different as it supports your own pancreas. It does not need to be taken with meals.

CLA, chromium and exercise are also very effective in reducing high blood sugar levels.

As an added incentive to eliminate sugar, please bear in mind some diabetes complications – heart disease and stroke, kidney disease, eye complications, oral health complications, damage to the nerves that run throughout the body, foot complications, skin complications, depression, amputation etc.

The chapters on Enzymes and Glandulars offer some help in normalizing the body and thus eliminating sugar cravings.

DIARRHEA – improper or tainted food, parasites, or a whole list of causes - homeopathic remedy Podophyllum

EPILEPSY – has many causes, low oxygen during birth, head injuries, brain tumors, infection, stroke, genetic conditions, abnormal levels of sodium or blood sugar. You should see a medical doctor for this ailment. In some cases, however, it can be caused by a magnesium deficiency. MegaFood has a plain food based magnesium tablet that is relatively easy to take but be cautious to take a food based calcium with magnesium in a ratio of 1/1 which usually requires taking an extra magnesium tablet.

Some natural remedies would be magnesium, extra sleep, no alcohol or caffeine, B vitamins, omega 3 and vitamin D.

EYESIGHT - I personally know of only one person over the age of 50 who does not wear corrective lenses and/or has not had corrective vision surgery. That person would be me. Decades ago I was given glasses to wear by an eye doctor for a mild astigmatism and found to my horror that whenever I removed the glasses, my vision had declined. I had to recover from wearing them to see normally. Well, that was the end of the glasses, think I threw them out.

Nearsightedness and farsightedness is actually a loss of the original curve of one's eyeball. And it can be regained if your vision is not too distorted, you probably can regain some or all of your normal vision.

There are books on line that give exercises to strengthen your eyes. One I know of is "Better Eyesight Regardless Of Age" by Patricia Bragg. These can be very helpful. Another must, and a supplement I personally take, is cod liver oil. Likewise, an essential fatty acids formula is therapeutic for the eyes. Both formulas come in capsules and liquid.

 One thing I have noticed with age is that I require somewhat more light to read. I use natural full spectrum lighting whenever possible. There is one natural lighting company that leads the rest. The Ott Lighting Company ottlite.com is the only one I personally would recommend. This natural lighting really saves one's eyes and is very helpful against the "winter blues" when the days are shorter. They have quite a selection of compact and regular fluorescent bulbs, as well as desk lamps, etc. They have an "instant on" feature not like some other compacts that have to hear up before they are at their full wattage capacity.

Now here's the key, find an optometrist or ophthalmologist who will work with you and give you a prescription one level lower than your regular prescription for you to wear as your eyes improve. By wearing your normal prescription glasses you weaken your eyes so that they never improve.

It's a step down procedure, strengthen your eyes with exercise and nutrition, step down to a lower prescription, strengthen your eyes with exercise and nutrition then step down to an even lower prescription.

Warning: Do not discard your eyeglasses or contact lenses, drive a vehicle or operate machinery without your glasses. This is dangerous as well as against the law.

HEART HEALTH – Krill oil for omega-3 fatty acids and CoQ10 in the ubiquinol form, in addition to a heart glandular.

HEARING – Sometimes a loss of hearing can be as simple as a build up of wax in one's ears. Instead of going to the ear doctor and having water blasted into your ear canal, the following alternative is suggested – it's called "ear candling". This is usually performed at an establishment where they offer body massages but inquire first.

The procedure is very simple. You lie on your side while a coned waxed candle is place in your ear after being inserted into a paper plate to catch the 'burn off' from the candle. The candle is then lit and the heat creates a suction that pulls the wax from your ear. At the end of each candle it can be opened to reveal just how much wax has been removed. You'll be amazed!

Realistically, you should have 3 candles for each ear as the wax buildup is rarely removed with just one candle. However, if you have this done regularly, 2 candles for each ear should suffice.

Once you see how this is done you can probably do this with the help of a responsible friend. DO NOT ATTEMPT THIS BY YOURSELF.

Most people have reported a noticeable increase in their hearing, however, if you still require improvement in your hearing, you should visit an ear specialist.

HICCUPS – are very annoying but prolonged hiccupping should have medical attention. I have found that if I'm lying on the couch having a snack, they can be more frequent. Here's my remedy – sit upright, stick your tongue out as far as you can while putting your index fingers in both your ears. At the same time push your abdomen forward and hold your breath. 30 seconds of this should do the trick. Honestly, I am not kidding, this works for me usually on the first try. If you are out in public, it might be wise to go to the rest room.

Another remedy is to put pressure under both eyebrows with your thumbs. This gets the vagus nerve involved and can short circuit the hiccups.

HIV – this nasty virus has eluded all attempts to kill it. The best one can do is stop it in its tract by suppressing it. Since most virus replicate every 12 hours, a twice a day treatment is needed. The natural product I know of that will accomplish this is Lomatium Isolate by Eclectic (the alcohol version). Truthfully, I have never used this product on a human but did rescue a cat who turned out to have feline aids, the feline counterpart of HIV.

She has been on the Lomatium Isolate for many years and is thriving. Once I decided to try an alternative and she became ill without the Lomatium. A few drops are added to plain water and taken orally. With the cat I use 1 drop in 1 oz. water and administer with a syringe orally (without the needle). The Reference Guild at the back of this book will tell you where to purchase.

INDIGESTION - As we age our ability to digest food diminishes. This explains all the acid reflux heartburn, and digestive problems experienced in this country. Before you run for the antacids, especially the over the counter drugs, know that these products impair one's ability to digest even more and compound the problem because the food is not being digested properly while valuable nutrients are not being absorbed by the body. This has severe consequences leading to malfunctions on every level.

THE SOLUTION FOR THIS IS SIMPLY TO TAKE A DIGESTIVE ENZYME CAPSULE WITH EVERY MEAL – not necessary if you are having a salad, fruit, or anything raw as they have their own enzymes. The chapter on Enzymes goes into much greater detail on this.

Too much protein creates an excess of acidity in the body. The kidneys need to buffer the acidic waste products before they can be excreted in the urine. This buffering is accomplished with calcium and if there is not enough calcium circulating in the bloodstream, it is pulled from the bone. The way around this is to take a calcium magnesium supplement just before eating a heavy or moderate meat meal.

Taking a probiotic supplement (this is different from a digestive enzyme) 40 minutes before a meal at least once a day will go a long way toward enhancing your immune system, assisting in adrenal hormone production, REDUCING CHOLESTEROL, and keeping all your hormones in balance. PROBIOTICS MUST BE TAKEN ON AN EMPTY STOMACH WITH NO FOOD FOR AT LEAST 30 MINUTES AFTERWARD. When taken with food, the digestive acids in your stomach destroys them.

A footnote here, both your appendix and your gallbladder play significant roles in digestion. If you are not in an acute life or death situation, it's best to explore natural ways to eliminate the inflammation and/or stones without removing the stones and/or the gallbladder. I know of people who have accomplished this.

INSOMNIA- this can be the result of side effects of a drug or drugs or too many cell towers near your residence or work place. See <u>antennasearch.</u> <u>com</u> and click on "towers". Deep Sleep by Herbs Etc. can help as well as more time outdoors needed, exercise.

INTESTINAL POISONS - are characterized by bad breath, body odor, putrid gas, digestive disorders, acne, prostate disorders, liver dysfunction, multiple allergic response syndrome (MARS), sluggish lymphatic system, multiple food allergies. Taking a bowel cleanser along with a probiotic (taken on an empty stomach), increasing fiber, and eliminating white flour and white sugar will go a long way in clearing up these problems.

KIDNEY PROBLEMS – cutting back on your salt intake will help save your kidneys. Please see the chapter on Salt - How Bad Is It?. Also, drinking extra distilled water from a home water distiller will help flush out any hardened non organic deposits. Finally, a kidney glandular will help support your kidneys. Warning: if your kidneys are totally non functioning, you will need dialysis and ultimately a transplant.

LIVER PROBLEMS- this calls for cutting back on alcohol consumption and red meat, while eliminating fried and fatty foods. Medications put a real strain on the liver, seek the natural remedies for the symptoms that are not life threatening.

Finally, I use Quantum's Liver Gallbladder Extract with alcohol. It comes in a non alcoholic version but I don't think it is as strong.

MEMORY – DNA complex, phosphatidyl serine DHA, Mental Sharp by Pure Encapsulations, Krill Oil, check for presence of mold in the home.

MENOPAUSE – Please see chapter For Women Only.

MIGRANE HEADACHES – can be caused by a toxic liver, consequently, medications that are given routinely over a period of time can actually stress the liver more and add to the problem. Liver Gallbladder Extract from Quantum can be very therapeutic.

OSTEOPOROSIS - Osteoporosis or thinning of the bones in the body most of the time is caused by the changing ratio of estrogen to progesterone usually after menopause where one's progesterone level drops to almost zero. This is explained in much more detail in the chapter For Women Only. The right progesterone cream can actually build bone.

Some additional facts on building or losing bone: For calcium to be incorporated into bone it requires enzymes, B6 and magnesium (in a 1:1 ratio with calcium) as catalysts. Vitamins A and E are also needed.

Excess phosphorus decreases calcium in bone, large amounts of potassium are antagonistic to magnesium. Soda contains phosphorus and enough of it will cause calcium to leach from one's bones.

A craving for chocolate is a sign of magnesium deficiency.

Vitamin K is helpful in bone building but needs to be used carefully as it causes the blood to thicken and clot. Persons using blood thinners should avoid this vitamin.

Eating large quantities of meat will result in calcium loss from bones as the result of a negative calcium balance which will pull calcium from the bones.

Persons who have used cortisone over a long period of time developed osteoporosis.

One of the first indications of osteoporosis is a loss of height.

X-rays show osteoporosis only when 30% of bone is lost.

1992 Journal of Orthopedics had a study on progesterone that showed 1 ½% bone loss per year of post menopausal women. Studies have shown that transdermal (topical) progesterone cream actually increases bone. But beware imitations.

PARASITES – there are many remedies out there to rid the body of, but I have recently discovered food grade diatomaceous earth, a powder that can be put in juice or any other liquid. CAUTION; THIS PRODUCT SHOULD NOT BE INHALED.

This powder strips the parasites of their exoskeltons (outer shell) and they die. To the best of my knowledge there are no side effects. This product should be taken long enough so that the life cycle of the "bug" does not produce offspring (approximately 35-45 days). And yes, it is thought that at least 90% of the human population has parasites.

PROSTATE PROBLEMS – the herb saw palmetto can be helpful. See chapter For Men Only

SKIN PROBLEMS – try a thorough bowel cleansing to rid the body of the toxins that are manifesting through eruptions and itching of the skin (Intestinal Cleansing Formula by Quantum Herbals. Also, a liver cleanse in addition can be of added benefit. The drugs prescribed for various skin conditions have some of the worst side effects known to man.

SKIN INFECTIONS – Goldline Ichthammol Ointment 20% is a very good black drawing save for topical infections. This should not be used for the mouth, ears, eyes or throat or any place internal.

TRANSPLANTS - Transplants should really be done as a last resort. It's not as simple replacing a spare part in your car. Your body does not want this organ/tissue from another person. It wants its own genetic material and goes to great lengths to reject this foreign body. It has been programmed to do so.

To get around this rejection doctors have to depress one's immune system to the point where the person needs to be monitored very closely in order to survive.

These anti-rejection drugs affect your entire body. Here are some side effects of transplants depending on which medication one is taking:

Nausea and vomiting

Headache

High blood pressure

High cholesterol

Puffy face

Anemia

Arthritis

Weakened bones

Increased appetite

Weight gain

Trouble sleeping

Mood swings

Swelling and tingling of the hands and feet

Tremors

Hair loss or unwanted hair growth

If your conditions is not severe, you might try supporting the affected organ with a corresponding glandular, while making sure your diet is free of refined foods. Please see chapter on Glandulars

TUMORS- are the result of an imbalance in the body. They are cells gone wild and growing where they don't belong. Enzyme therapy has been known to banish tumors but this gets a little tricky. If you have a slow growing tumor where you can take a month to see if your tumor is shrinking from the enzymes, fine. However, if you have a monster growing at the speed of light, medical intervention is necessary.

The Medizym systemic enzyme is taken on an empty stomach with no food for at least 45 minutes afterward. This ensures that stomach acids will not penetrate the enteric coating around the tablet and destroy its effectiveness.

Also, digestive enzymes should be taken with every meal, at the end of the meal. These are a different type of enzyme designed to be taken with food.

Finding a medical practitioner who is familiar with this type of treatment will be very helpful. Again, eliminate white sugar and white flour.

ULCERS – Gastro Pro by Progressive Labs boasts a product with specific natural ingredients to alleviate symptoms of ulcers and gastro-intestinal disorders.

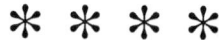

CHAPTER 13
Glandular Therapy

Glandular therapy is the use of whole animal glands for health maintenance and of health problems usually involving malfunctioning organs in the body. For example, liver glandulars benefit and support the liver, while kidney glandulars support the kidneys, etc.

Studies have shown that animals with damaged livers had liver regeneration after being administered liver glandulars, the same with the thyroid gland, etc.

These glandular supplements may also provide nutrients and hormones in a low dose form, in addition to improved digestion which improves overall health.

Common Uses Of Glandular Therapy

Thyroid, adrenal, heart, liver, kidney, neurologic diseases, diabetes, pancreatic insufficiency, urinary incontinence, and thymus for immune disorders.

Because these supplements are relatively concentrated it is very important to use ORGANIC glandulars whenever possible. Progressive Labs also has an extensive line of glandulars. ' Like heals like' is the prevailing theory.

An ovarian glandular is for female support of the ovaries, while the male glandular equivalent will contain orchic (testicle) concentrate (more pedal to the metal).

As a precaution, I understand there can be some mild allergic reactions although I have never experienced any or known of anyone who has.

Please keep in mind this same therapy has been used successfully in humans and our pets are now benefiting from the technology as well.

Glandulars I take for organ support

Ovary – Solaray Female Caps 2/day

Pituitary – Progressive Labs 1/day

Adrenal – Nutricology 1/day, also available from Progressive Labs

Thyroid – Nutricology 1/day, also available from Progressive Labs

Note: If your thyroid is normal, you probably don't need a thyroid glandular, mine is a little sluggish

* * * *

CHAPTER 14
Weight Gain/Loss

First of all, you have to be emotionally ready to lose weight. If you are eating to console yourself for a loss, depression or lack of self esteem, the chances of your losing weight are stacked against you. You can tell that you are eating emotionally if you're eating when you are not hungry or eating when you are depressed. Granted there is a lot in this world to be depressed about, but instead of drowning your sorrows with food, it might be wise to seek counseling, either with a friend or a professional,

Next you need to get the 'bad stuff' out of the house. Don't bring it through the front door. If it's bad for you, it's bad for your children and will have serious consequences for everyone sooner or later. In this book we will attempt to learn some healthier tasty alternatives, but the sooner you and your children start eating properly, the better.

When you are older and sometimes sooner, your fat tends to accumulate on your abdomen and hips and is much harder to lose.

Fat cells have memory and when you have them in excess, losing weight only makes them shrink, not decrease in numbers. They hang out waiting for the opportunity to plump back up. Liposuction is the only thing that will get rid of their numbers, but for some reason this causes a shifting of fat cells in some, if not in most people, to another part of the body. For instance, if you have liposuction on your abdomen, you may experience a fat shift to your hips or thighs.

As a scientist, here is something I have learned. There are finger like projections in our colons attached to the wall of the intestine called 'villi' which collect nutrients and channel them into our bodies. Eating the wrong foods causes these 'villi' to get clogged and become impacted. This severely impedes nutrient absorption and when the brain does not get the signal that it has received the nutrients, it triggers a hunger response for more food. We eat more food in response to the 'hunger call' and end up eating more calories that we really need which translate to added weight most of the time. Weight loss supplements ultimately fail because of this process.

Also, the lack of enzymes in the food put a large burden on our systems for digestion. Taking a digestive enzyme with meals is a must for persons over 40.

Drastically reducing calories reduces the body's metabolic activity – the ability to burn off fat – by reducing thyroid activity.

How do we correct this situation? The first and best way is prevention. The main culprits in this scenario are white flour, white sugar, and lack of fiber.

This requires a commitment to read food labels diligently.

Let's examine white flour as an ingredient. If the label reads 'enriched', this means that the manufacturers have taken whole grain and stripped it of all its nutrients and have added back a small amount of those nutrients back. Of course, once those nutrients have been tampered with, they will never be in the same state or quantity as in the original state.

If the label reads "wheat flour", this is still white flour with as little as a pinch of whole wheat flour added. The amount of whole wheat flour added is strictly at the discretion of the "manufacturer, but as little as a few grains makes it legal for them to call it 'wheat flour". The label should read 'whole wheat flour' or 'whole grain' and name the grain or grains. Many years ago school children used to use white flour and water as glue for their art projects. This combination works the same way in our intestines and makes a sticky glue in our intestines.

White sugar works in a slightly different way to sabotage us. In addition to having the brain signal for more nutrients, it specifically signals for more sugar and throws our insulin levels into overdrive so that our bodies ultimately crash. The way the body compensates is to ask for more sugar to restore energy. Very few people can consume large quantities of sugar and not gain weight. If the label reads sorbitol or any other ingredient ending in 'ol' or 'ose' as in sucrose or fructose. This is a back door way to put sugar into the product without being obvious. Refined sugar in any form paves the way for diabetes. The product should read "unrefined cane sugar", fruit juice sweetened, agave, or stevia to be the real deal.

I have recently heard television advertising stating "all sugars are the same". Basically, this is true, but it's what happens to the sugar after it is harvested is the key. Some sugars are left in their natural unrefined state which is just what our bodies require, but most sugars are taken and refined in many forms such as fructose, corn syrup, etc.

Foods with fiber are very helpful in losing weight. The fiber we need on a daily basis should be around 25 grams to keep our bowels functioning smoothly. This requires you to read the labels and get into the habit of keeping track of how much fiber we are ingesting on a daily basis. After a while you will know by memory the fiber content of the foods you eat routinely.

Also, as little as 2 weeks of vitamin A deficiency may reduce thyroid hormone secretion significantly (the gland that helps to regulate your weight). A B2 (riboflavin) deficiency may also depress the thyroid by reducing the amount of hormones it secretes. A B6 (pyridoxine) deficiency will also depressed thyroid function by reducing the conversion of iodine into thyroid hormones. Poor thyroid functioning may also cause a decrease in the utilization of vitamin B12, a vitamin necessary for forming nucleic acids DNA and RNA . These acids are necessary for fat, carbohydrate and protein metabolism.

GTF chromium optimizes the metabolism of carbohydrates. Since this is deficient in people who eat too many refined foods, it would be wise to take a daily supplement of this mineral.

If all this sounds like a lot of trouble, I can assure you it's worth it. It is unfortunate that we live in a society where the emphasis is on the junk food. By junk food I mean food that has been tampered with one way or another and is not in its original state, thereby having an adverse effect on one's body.

Shopping at a health food store and/or a supermarket that carries organic food is a must. Let me address a misconception about real food. It's true that most organic and whole foods may cost a little more, but consider this- because these whole foods enter the body in a more perfect state, they satisfy your appetite faster and for a longer period of time, thus you require less food and the overall cost may be the same or less. The whole foods are simply more filling and certainly are better for you. Starchy while flour products may be filling at first, but ultimately they produce cravings for more calories long before eating a whole food meal would.

An intestinal cleanser is a quick way to clean out your system and lose a few pounds. To get rid of the accumulated waste in the bowel I would recommend a gentle 'roto rooter' called Cleanse Blend by Premier. One teaspoon in juice once a day has a very positive effect on drawing out the toxins and freeing up the 'villi'. It also comes in capsules, but the powder is more cost effective. I have found that it reduces my appetite as well. Quantum also makes a very effective intestinal cleanser in 2 parts. Part 1 is a capsule, followed by part 2 which is a powder taken in juice.

Something else to try may be a pituitary glandular if you are over 40. Most people over 50 have a very sluggish pituitary as a consequence of the aging process. The pituitary is the 'master gland' that controls all the other organs. It has a positive effect on weight metabolism.

Some additional obstacles to weight loss: liver malfunction, thyroid malfunction, lack of correct supplements, and hormone imbalance. Please note: one should have a thyroid profile blood test to determine if one's thyroid is malfunctioning.

Please see Chapters on Glandulars and Joan's Picks.

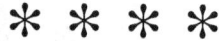

CHAPTER 15
The 24 Hour Fast

Fasting is something that should be undertaken under the supervision of a trained professional, only if you have no issues such as diabetes, low blood sugar, etc that would preclude fasting. Here is a simple way to try a very short 24 hour short fast. DURING THIS SHORT FAST YOU ARE ALLOWED, AND EVEN ENCOURAGED TO DRINK AS MUCH SPRING OR DISTILLED WATER AS YOU WOULD LIKE (distilled water should not be from a plastic bottle as the plastic leaches into the water (distilled water has osmotic properties).

Your body may give you a hard time about fasting so pick a day when your work load is minimal such as a Sunday. Upon awakening drink a large glass of water then try not to think about food. Stay out of the kitchen! See how long you last before the hunger pains and/or weakness bring you to your limit. Then try a 6 oz glass of organic unsweetened juice (preferable apple) to stave off hunger. When the hunger returns, try another glass of juice.

The aim here is to make it to dinner without eating. Don't be discouraged if you fail the first or second time. Your body needs to get used to the idea of going a little longer without food. A second attempt can be tried a few days later depending upon how you feel.

Here's what this 24 hour fast will accomplish. First, it actually has the effect of shrinking your stomach somewhat – sort of a mini gastric bypass without any of the surgery. Some weight loss is usually a side effect of this method. Second, it starts to cleanse your body of nasty toxins. Third, it sharpens your taste buds and makes you aware of excess sweeteners and salt. Your food can actually taste better and your sense smell and hearing can increase.

Using this method once a week will maximize your health greatly. You should find that each time you attempt this fast you can go longer and longer before eating.

A word of caution – some persons have a natural ability to fast for several days feeling very little discomfort while others have to be very careful dealing with the possibility of dizziness and weakness. After 36 hours you really should have a health professional monitor you as too many toxins being released at the same time can be harmful. If at any time you feel extremely weak, you should abandon the fast.

When resuming eating you should start off with some juice, wait a while then eat very lightly with small portions excluding heavy proteins such as red meat. Longer fasts have an actual protocol on how to resume eating which you can probably download off the internet in addition to many books on how to fast.

Mother often said "if you don't eat, you'll get sick". The problem is that too many wrong foods HAVE MADE US SICK.

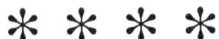

CHAPTER 16
Vitamins Anyone?

As far as I'm concerned, there are only 2 types of vitamins manufactured – 'food' and 'fake'. The fake vitamins are simply synthetic ingredients which are formulated in such a way as to be of no use to the human body, in fact they actually conflict with the body's natural functions. Why? Because they originate from unnatural sources and then are heated as to destroy any possible remaining benefits they might have had. Just because the bottle says "vitamin" on the label does not mean it is a healthy supplement.

A good way to prove which vitamins are compatible with your body is by holding the vitamin bottle in one hand and outstretching your other arm horizontally out to your side. Then have a friend to push down on your \ outstretched arm while you attempt to resist. If your arm goes down very readily, this is the wrong vitamin or supplement for your body.

You will find that with most whole food vitamins your arm should stay outstretched in spite of the external pressure to push it down. This is simply because it is natural and is compatible with your body.

Then there are the "knock off" vitamins that are manufactured with packaging that mimics the real deal. A clue here is price – very rarely can a quality product be offered for "half price". If it walks and talks like a duck, it probably is a duck, not a vitamin.

Whole food vitamin manufacturers are few and far between – MegaFood is the only real whole food vitamin manufacturer with cold fusion that I know of.

For example, vitamin E should be a complex of alpha, beta, gamma and delta E along with their corresponding tocotrienols. Just plain d'alpha E is an incomplete formula, dl'alpha (with the "l" added) means it is a synthetic formula

ORDERING VITAMINS AND SUPPLEMENTS ON LINE

Most natural vitamin supplements should not be exposed to high heat therefore it is prudent to take the summer heat into account when ordering.

But what is more important is 'how' your package is shipped. The use of gamma ray emitters is now being used by the Post Office and Federal Express to scan the contents of packages. I presume they are looking for explosives or who knows what.

THIS HIGH ENERCY IONIZING GAMMA RADAITION CAN DESTROY NUTRITIONAL SUPPLEMENTS. These gamma rays are produced by radioactive elements such as radium and are highly toxic. Not only do these rays neutralize the supplements, but it is unknown as to how the changes in the nutrient's molecular structure affect the human body. You can bet it's not an improvement and is detrimental.

Needless to say, your vitamins will no longer be viable and compatible with your body and may even be harmful if ingested. In short, all nutrients will be destroyed.

The only shipping company I know of who does not scan with gamma rays is UPS who virtually guarantees no irradiation. Do not confuse United Parcel Service (UPS) with United States Post Office (USPS) who does irradiate. Not all packages are scanned but how will you know?

Now a word about on line suppliers. Some companies buy a large quantity of supplements from the vitamin manufacturer in order to offer a better price. While there is nothing wrong with this, you need to find out how the product was shipped to them and, of course, how they will be shipping it to you, as well as the length of time they have warehoused the product and at what temperature.

I recently was in the process of purchasing an item from a distributor of a vitamin company when I found out that the parent company was mailing their products to their distributor via Fed Express and subsequently mailing me the product via the post office. This was potentially a double dose of gamma radiation. I immediately started ordering directly from the company that ships UPS (the good guys) to its consumers.

Reputable companies only ship via UPS when they become aware of the problem. One company I know of will not accept a return unless it is shipped back via UPS. This way they don't put a damaged product back in stock. Kudos to them.

In conclusion, when buying on line, you really don't know what has happened to a product and where it has been stored (possibly a hot warehouse for weeks or even months) , however, if you are determined to save a few pennies, you might as well just take your money and throw it in the street. It's the same difference because once a nutrient is damaged, it becomes toxic to the body and you are better off not taking it.

Please see chapter "Joan's Picks" and the Reference Guide at the back of this book.

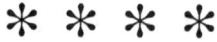

CHAPTER 17
For Women Only

Husbands and boyfriends should read this chapter as well. It's time that we drastically changed our thinking with reference to women's health.

Let's start with the big "C", breast cancer, uterine cancer, ovarian cancer, cervical cancer. For decades we've been told to be on the lookout for lumps, bleeding, irregular menstrual cycles, etc. and if cancer should be discovered by one's doctor, we should take immediate steps toward chemotherapy, surgery, and/or radiation. Some women live in such fear of breast cancer as to have their perfectly normal breasts removed. No thank you!

The medical protocol was to have a mammogram once a year to screen for breast cancer (they have now changed this recommendation to once every other year because of the radiation factor). With my family history of both a mother and maternal grandmother having had breast cancer it would seem that I would be a very high risk. But with the prevention protocol I employ I can state that I have never had a mammogram or breast cancer. If I had followed the medical protocol and had yearly mammograms after age 40, to date my body would have endured 27 "grams" and, in my opinion, my risk of breast cancer would have increased significantly.

The following information may seem a little bit 'off the wall', but a medical doctor actually has proven the following. Female cancers thrive in an estrogen dominate environment. This occurs when the estrogen is out of balance with the other hormones in a woman's body and becomes dominate. When this happens, tissues can proliferate and form tumors.

The solution is easier than you think, simply use a topical progesterone cream twice a day every day with 5 days off every month. which will put the estrogen back in balance. Dr. John Lee conducted a study of 356 women with breast cancer with the progesterone cream treatment and had a 100 PER CENT CURE RATE.

With the estrogen back in balance the tumors could not survive and dissolved on their own without any medical intervention.

Another bonus from this cream is that is can actually stop cancer from forming in the first place. I have not been privileged to conduct my own case studies, but I can tell you that after years of using this cream cancer has not knocked on my door especially since my past history included a bad pap when I was in my 30's (way before I knew about progesterone cream).

Here are some ailments associated with a progesterone DEFICIENCY:

Mood swings, breast tenderness, decreased sex drive, depression, insomnia, irritability, anxiety, weight gain, fatigue, headaches and migraines, hot flashes, blood sugar disorders, inability to concentrate, memory loss irregular menstrual periods and/or heavy prolonged periods.

About 18 months ago I decided to go to a female GYN for a check up. She asked me how long it had been since my last exam to which I replied, "about 10 years". The surprised look on her face after the exam indicated that she had thought that after since so much time had elapsed that she would certainly discover something irregular yet she could find no evidence of anything out of the ordinary. Patients like me are not good for business but my role in life is not to get sick to support the medical profession.

Now for the side effects of this progesterone cream. First of all it can promote a youthful appearance. Your body likes being in balance and may reward you accordingly in your mirror.

Second, with your body more in sync you can also notice an increase in your libido (sex drive).

Third, it reduces or can even eliminate 'hot flashes' associated with menopause. Another helpful product to banish hot flashes is an ovarian glandular. (Please see chapter on Glandulars).

Fourth, it has been proven to increase bone density significantly to help eliminate osteoporosis. This is much better than some prescriptions that can wreck havoc with your liver and actually cause bone breakage.

And, of course, fifth, your chances of getting a female type cancer are greatly diminished. Nothing is an absolute guarantee, especially if you have an improper diet, but I live a cancer free life and would like all women to explore this possibility.

This is such an important item that I've added a link to my web site joanyork.com – the cost is $24.95 for the 2 oz. jar and $34.95 for the 3 oz pump. In my opinion, the Feminine Balance Therapy formula works best for women under the age of 45 while the Balance Plus Therapy which has some phytoestrogens added, works best for women over 45.

Not all brands are alike, therefore, this is the one endorsed by Dr. Lee.

Compare this to the standard medical approach for hot flashes which is to prescribe MORE estrogen. Giving estrogen increases one's risk of cancer hence the warning on the label and the limited length of time one should take this hormone. If this sounds backwards, it is just that. If you lose your balance, you will fall down and if your body loses its chemical or hormonal balance, you will fall into some form of disease. It's the law of cause and effect.

Speaking of hormones there is a birth control product on the market that causes one's body to have only 4 menstrual cycles a year instead of the NORMAL 12. Our bodies were designed to have monthly periods and to tamper with our body's balance with imbalanced doses of hormones is just asking for trouble. I know of one person who tried this product and had to stop taking it immediately. She didn't give me all the reasons. For the record, the monthly shedding of the uterine wall cleanses the body of toxins and promotes a clean environment for conception.

Menopause - I have never met a woman nearing menopause who was wishing for her periods to continue. Having postponed menopause for as long as I could (age 57), I can testify that the side effects of menopause are true. This is expressly why I take supplements that basically tell my body I'm not as old as the calendar says, specifically and ovarian glandular, a pituitary glandular, and progesterone cream (topically).

Some side effects of menopause are the loss of the laying down of new bone, loss of waistline, weight gain around one's midsection, diminished sex drive, loss of muscle tone with sagging skin, loss of hormones causing hormone imbalance and skin wrinkling (people are amazed that I don't have wrinkles, except for some fine ones more visible with a magnifying glass), See joanyork.com "The Calendar Lies, Believe Your Eyes".

Women experience heart attacks several years after menopause mainly due to arterial spasms rather than a build up of plaque in the arteries. This is related to a severe drop in progesterone levels which causes the arterial walls to spasm. If the spasm lasts long enough, blood supply is cut off to the heart and death results. HRT'S have not been proven to help the heart in any way and have quite a few nasty side effects including caner, double vision, severe abdominal pain, severe mental depression, loss of appetite, etc.

Again, the progesterone cream mentioned earlier in this chapter should be very helpful in relieving hot flashes from menopause. Another helpful product to help banish hot flashes is an ovarian glandular. Please see chapter on Glandulars.

✳ ✳ ✳ ✳

CHAPTER 18
Pregnancy

Let's start with health before, during and after pregnancy. All too many women start their pregnancies in poor health and inadequate nutrition. By this I mean that knowingly or unknowingly their bodies do not have the nutrition to support a fetus properly. The fetus will take as much nutrition as he can from the mother which puts the mother in even worse health. This is complicated further during future pregnancies which could end in a miscarriage for this very reason. This lack of nutrition will manifest itself in the health of the baby and have an impact on his/her development.

Likewise, a significant portion of women begin their pregnancies when they are considerably overweight, some even morbidly obese. Without proper nutrition the way is paved for birth defects and unhealthy babies. Unless there is a defective gene involved, I believe most birth defects are a direct result of improper diet and drugs. If you doubt this, read a book on 'embryology' and discover just how intricate the steps are in the development of the baby. It's simply mild boggling. Without the proper nutritional components from the mother things are bound to go wrong. Even if you are fortunate enough to escape birth defects, you may have a child who is predisposed to being overweight or have other health problems his/her entire life.

As stated earlier, fat cells have memory and when you have them in excess, losing weight only makes them shrink, not decrease in numbers. They hang out waiting for the opportunity to plump back up. Liposuction is the only thing that will get rid of their numbers, but for some reason this causes a shifting of fat cells in some, if not in most people, to another part of the body. For instance, if you have liposuction on your abdomen, you may experience a fat shift to your hips or thighs.

In short, the only way to optimize your chances of a healthy baby is to have optimum nutrition for several months, if not at least a year, before becoming pregnant, during the pregnancy and certainly thereafter. For instance, a B12 vitamin deficiency in expectant mothers may increase the risk of crying babies. Also, living near power lines and long daily exposure to electromagnetic fields such as cell phone or computers has been linked to premature births, low birth weights and miscarriages.

AN INCREASE IN HEALTHY CHILDREN AND THEIR MOTHERS WILL SAVE UNTOLD BILLIONS IN HEALTH CARE.

Have you seen the advertisements on TV for attorneys wanting to represent women who took certain drugs during their pregnancy and had children with birth defects? Taking drugs during a pregnancy is flirting with disaster and should be avoided unless there is some life threatening emergency.

For women who have trouble becoming pregnant due to a hormone imbalance, the addition of a topical progesterone cream can help considerably. Please see the Reference Index on where to purchase and the chapters For Women Only and Harmful Electromagnetic Fields.

And now a possible cure for "morning sickness"? Apparently the new baby on board causes a decrease in one's trace minerals. Taking a trace mineral supplement can take care of the nausea. Be advised though, you need to purchase a separate trace mineral supplement for extra potency not just a vitamin that has trace minerals as part of the formula.

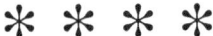

CHAPTER 19
For Men Only

In this country Viagra sales are off the charts which clearly indicates men experience some form of "performance" issues. Drugs for this problem promote blood flow to the lower region but in some cases the constricted blood vessels do not return to normal. In the case of an erection which does not subside, medical intervention is clearly indicated. The pain being experienced means that some tissue is dying which can lead to the permanent loss of the ability to have an erection if enough tissue is destroyed.

This constriction of blood vessels can also cut off circulation to the optic nerve and cause permanent blindness if one has a tight bundling of blood vessels and nerves in the small space in the back of the eyes.

Here are some possible causes of this dysfunction along with a few suggestions:

Low testosterone – it is perfectly normal for a man's testosterone levels to drop as one gets older. This can be treated medically with hormone injections if one's "T" values are EXTREMELY low. However, a more natural approach would be an orchic glandular extracted from bovine testicles. The glandular supports the part of the body that needs help. I use an ovarian glandular and it works wonders, the orchic glandular is the male counterpart. Progressive Labs makes this product under the name "Androzyme". The reference guide at the back of this book tells how to contact them along with a 20% discount upon mention of this book.

Also, olive oil is reported to increase testosterone but I suspect not to the same level of the orchic glandlular.

Low sperm count – has been reported in connection with excessive exposure to electromagnetic fields such as heavy cell phone and computer usage and/or living in close proximity to power lines (closer than 1200 feet). Please see chapter on Harmful Electromagnetic Fields.

Weight gain – one's body is having trouble with circulation due to all those extra pounds. Please see the chapters on Weight Loss and The Disease Of Denial.

In a European study SPET-085, an ethanol extract of saw palmetto was found to be as effective as finasteride, the standard prescription drug used in blocking the enzyme that leads to benign prostatic hyperploasia (BPH). Most side effects are rare, however, saw palmetto is being marketed on the internet as a remedy to grow hair on balding heads or at least stop any future baldness. That's a side effect most men may want.

Psychological – for openers this would require talking to someone who will listen to you, whether it is a friend or professional. It's best to get to the root of the problem. Also, it's a very bad idea for either or both partners to "let themselves go" physically, bad for one's health and self esteem.

Penile length – there is actually a minor surgical operation (phalloplasty) that involves surgically releasing a certain muscle at the base of the penis that allows more of it to be exposed. Before you run off to the doctor, it is my understanding that the length gained usually can be up to 1-2 inches but no more than that.

Certainly select a doctor who does this operation at least somewhat routinely, not someone who has to look it up in a book. Also, this procedure most likely could be done without a general anesthetic, ask if it could be done with a local anesthetic. A general anesthetic is more money for the doctors but higher risk for you. This procedure takes 45 minutes to an hour.

There is also a procedure called "girth enhancement" whereby some Belladerm skin grafts are inserted into the penis to make it wider. This procedure takes approximately 2 1/2 hours and should be done with a general anesthetic but conceivably could be done with a local.

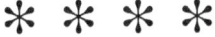

CHAPTER 20
Getting Rid Of Pain The Natural Way

Pain is the body's warning system that something is very wrong and needs to be dealt with. Pain medication deliberately stands in the way of the CAUSE OF THE PAIN being treated and the pain being eliminated. Most medications put a strain on the liver and divert it from its task of helping the body run smoothly by filtering out the day to day toxins.

There are basically 2 types of pain, acute and chronic. When acute pain hits, such as a tooth abscess, by all means run for the pain killers. Once you have the abscess treated, the medication will no longer be needed.

Chronic pain is a different story. Most of us are trained to get relief from the pain even if we know what is causing the pain. Living one's life on pain medication (other than a terminal disease or something major) can do more harm that good. Dealing with the cause of the pain on a natural level and thereby not needing any pain medication is a much better way to go.

Drug companies see it differently. They have no interest in your finding the cause of the problem. Their advertising emphasizes the relief you will receive from their product, without suggesting steps to address the root cause of the pain. Life is not a contest to see how much pain medication we can take before our bodies ultimately break down and stop working. Those side effects are real and dangerous, not something to fill up air time in their advertising campaigns.

A notable exception – if you are suffering from a chronic, terminal disease, it is the humane thing for a doctor to prescribe pain killers. HOWEVER, IF THE PAIN MEDICATION IS STANDING IN THE WAY OF DETERMINING EXACTLY WHAT IS CAUSING THE PAIN, IT SHOULD BE DISCONTINUED AND NATURAL REMEDIES EXPLORED WITH A DOCTOR WHO DEALS IN THESE REMEDIES.

Please be sure to get a diagnosis for your condition before attempting natural remedies. See chapters on Ailments and Diseases, and Enzymes.

Let's deal with 2 major pains that many people have –migraines and arthritis. First, most migraines are caused by an overworked or toxic liver. When one takes pain medication for the migraine, this overworks the liver even more. Ultimately, the migraines can increase in severity and frequency while one needs to increase the medication.

I decided to try out my theory on myself when confronted with only the third migraine I have ever had in my life. For the record this migraine was very painful, sensitive to light and noise .and generally incapacitating. I ran for some liver detox extract by Quantum (wonderful stuff to have on hand) and within 30 minutes the migraine was completely gone. Please bear in mind that I don't ingest caffeine nor was I on any other medication as migraines can be the direct result of caffeine or medication withdrawal.

Since the migraine incident I pay a lot more attention to my liver and now take a liver cleanse on a regular basis. For the record this migraine was huge, sensitive to light and noise and was generally incapacitating. I'm sure there are other causes of migraines, but I believe that liver involvement is responsible for a large percentage of them.

General - osteoarthritis with its accompanying pain occurs when the fluid in the joints lessens with age and the opposing bone cartilage starts having friction. If this problem is not dealt with, most people will end up becoming incapacitated or requiring a hip or knee replacement.

Here is where you need to be very careful. Since pain is the body's warning system, taking pain medication shuts off the body's warning system so that more damage is allowed to occur without any warning from the body. Then, after enough damage occurs and the cartilage is worn down, the limb becomes incapacitated and it's too late.

I've had arthritis in my right knee for many years from knee surgery in my teens. I suspect I've had some cartilage loss as well in the. A chicken cartilage supplement (1000 mg) and Glucosamine Chrondroitin (2 different products) taken daily give me nearly 100% of my knee's function and I am pain free most of the time. Major storms seem to make my knee twinge, but the pain is short lived and requires NO MEDICATION.

As an added bonus, you have no accumulation of medication in your liver which can eventually cause the liver to shut down. A friend of mine's husband had to have a liver transplant to prevent his death from cancer of his liver. Now he MUST take anti-rejection drugs which lower his immune system and make him susceptible to all types of diseases. In his case one of the consequences of a particular anti-rejection medication he was given was that he started having small strokes which stopped when the doctors changed his medication. He has no choice, he must stay on the medication for the rest of his probably shortened life.

One also has to be careful not to take any immune stimulants as they works against the medication and can lead to a rejection of the transplant.

Please see chapter on Ailments and Diseases..

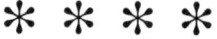

CHAPTER 21
Dental Secrets

Dental diseases can severely impact our overall general health. This may come as a surprise to some people but some fillings, crowns, bridge work, etc. can seriously affect your health depending on what materials are used. These substances are made from inorganic materials and can react with the body's tissues and cause illness and weakness.

To illustrate the point I know a dentist who practices natural dentistry who told me of a case of a woman who came to him feeling very ill. She had just had a new crown installed in her mouth and ever since had felt very sick. He tested her and found out that she was allergic to the materials in the crown and once it was removed she recovered completely. He subsequently fitted her with a crown made of materials she was not sensitive to and none of the negative symptoms reoccurred.

To this end a company called Biocomp Labs, 1621 North Circle Drive, Colorado Springs, Colorado NJ 80909. Phone – 1-719-548-1600 offers a blood test that tests the serum of one's blood against the many dental restoratives available and gives you a complete report of which materials you react to negatively (Highly Reactive) and the ones you don't react to (Least Reactive). You simply obtain a doctor or dentist's prescription to have your blood drawn at a private lab or at the doctor's office. The blood is then spun down then given back to you for mailing in a pre ordered mailer. Be sure to order the mailer first from Biocomp Labs in advance of the blood work as a delay in shipping could spoil the sample.

They will also provide you with a list of dentists in your area at their website who are familiar with this technology. Then you can take this report to your local dentist and request that he use only those materials that are "Least Reactive" on the report in your mouth. It's that easy.

However, this does not deal with restorations that have been inserted in your mouth prior to the report. It's up to you as to how much time, effort and money you wish to invest in replacements, but I can assure you any investment in your health pays big dividends.

A word about one of the most harmful substances you could put in your mouth in my opinion. Amalgam, (silver mercury) fillings give off a toxic gas when you chew which gets absorbed by the body. While this is at a relatively low level, long term exposure has suggested symptoms of hands, eyelids, or lips shaking. It may also cause headaches, trouble sleeping, personality change, birth defects, autoimmune disorders, neurodegenerative disease, memory loss, irritability, loss of intelligence, skin rash, sores in the mouth and/or sore and swollen gums. Reportedly these symptoms abate when the exposure is gone.

Sadly, many dentists still use silver fillings as it is cheaper and easier to use than composite fillings. It seems that the majority of these dentists past 60 years of age experience a diminished hand and eye coordination which is something to consider when choosing a dentist. You can always inquire over the phone "what year did doctor graduate?"

A dental story – several years ago I had some severe pain near a back molar and had visited several dentists each with a different specialty to determine the cause of the pain. This investigation lasted over a year as each dentist had a diagnosis based on his specialty. The periodontists each told me I needed a bone graft, the endodontists told me I needed a root canal procedure, and the general dentists who did not perform root canals or bone grafts told me I should extract the tooth. It turned out that root canal was the correct answer and the tooth was saved. So much for the age of specialization. This was years before my research on enzyme therapy. Today I would have it surgically drained if the antibiotics did not take care of the problem followed by a regime of immune strengthening enzyme therapy.

Extracting teeth causes many problems including bone loss with the adjacent teeth shifting at an angle on each side in toward the open space. Implants, I am told , have a propensity to attract bacteria inside the gum where the post is placed although I can't confirm this. Furthermore, most porcelain crowns and implants are composed of an aluminum compound which has a negative reaction with most, if not all, people's health. There is a diamond crown made of a plastic compound that is much more compatible with the body than the aluminum compound. This type of crown will not produce wear on any opposing teeth. Just don't crack walnuts in the shell with any crown. The life expectancy of this diamond type substance is around 20 years so it's a good contender especially for teeth near the front of one's mouth.

The moral of the story is simple – get a second opinion from a dentist with a different specialty. Likewise be wary of dentists who suggest grinding your tooth or teeth down to a stump and have a crown installed for any tooth that isn't perfect. Many times a composite filling will suffice but the profit on a crown vs. a filling is much greater for the dentist.

Recently I visited a dentist because I had a space between my upper 2 back teeth and was catching considerable food between these teeth. This is easily fixed by building out a composite filling on one of the teeth. However, he suggested I have both teeth outfitted with crowns. Outrageous!!! This would be a cost difference of $100-200, vs. thousands for the crowns and the loss of the natural enamel of 2 teeth. It has been my personal experience that crowns never fit the same way at the gum line, can cause irritation, and after a period of time need to be replaced. Also, if you must crown a tooth, be sure the metal at the base of the crown is not one you are "highly reactive" to on your compatibility report. These metals can be substituted for one that you have tested "least reactive" and as stated earlier, a "diamond" crown, not an aluminum one would be best as everyone is very reactive to aluminum.

Remember, most dentists recommendations are strongly connected to their wallets (at least the ones I know).

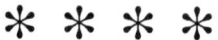

MEDICAL ISSUES

CHAPTER 22
You Gotta Be Kidding!!

We truly live in a brainwashed society regarding the use of prescription drugs. Let's take the case of someone who is suffering from depression. This is a very serious debilitating disease and it is no wonder that someone would overlook the major side effects of the prescription just to get some relief.

However, one must look at the overall picture. One of the major side effects of anti-depressant drugs is "DEPRESSION". "Thoughts of suicide" is also on the list of side effects.

One must assume that a large number of people taking these drugs are not experiencing the relief they require because there are secondary anti-depressant drugs to take in conjunction with the first anti-depressants. And guess what? These secondary drugs have many of the same side effects as the first ones only now there is double the chance of these very nasty side effects.

Also, patients with coronary artery disease taking commonly prescribed anti-depressants may be at significantly higher risk of death than those who are not taking these drugs.

You gotta be kidding!!

Warning: If you are currently on a life support drug such as insulin or have had a transplant you MUST CONTINUE to take your medication.

SOCIETY NEEDS TO KNOW HOW TO SOLVE THESE PROBLEMS WITHOUT DRUGS. As simple as this may sound, B complex vitamins have been known to have a very positive effect on the brain and depression and there have been some positive results with reference to schizophrenia. I prefer the Balanced B Complex from MegaFood which is food based and since it is water soluble, you can't overdose. Keep in mind, though, that B vitamins can have a diuretic effect and taking them in excess could lead to some minor dehydration.

And then there are the immune depressant drugs for autoimmune diseases such as rheumatoid arthritis, myasthenia gravis, lupus, Crohn's disease etc.

Autoimmune diseases occur when one's own immune system starts attacking one's body. The answer lies in finding out why this is happening, such as an imbalance in the system. Instead the method of treatment is to give medication to depress the immune system. This way the symptoms can be lessened. This does nothing to correct the problem and probably makes it worse. What this treatment does do is put the patient at risk for all types of other diseases that will attack a person with a weakened immune system. Personally I would avoid any drug where one possible side effect is "DEATH" or to put it more eloquently "FATAL EVENT".

One drug manufacturer strongly suggests (it may be mandatory) that you take a tuberculosis test before starting their drug. Chances are it will come back negative. Wonderful, but wait a minute!! One of the possible side effects of their drug IS TB! Are you kidding me? Not only that, but TB is quite contagious so you have the possibility of passing this disease on to your family, friends, hospital workers etc. As for the treatment for the TB, their drug has caused, take a guess. The treatment consists of a series of drugs for many months. Definitely a win, win for the drug companies, but not for YOUR health.

So we have another example of drugs which require other drugs to combat the side effects of the original drugs and possibly more drugs for the secondary drug's side effects. I recently heard a TV commercial where the husband stated that both he and his wife they were taking 12 prescriptions. I have heard of single individuals taking 20 or more prescriptions – this is just plain crazy when there are natural remedies that will do the job better than the harmful drugs.

Again, if you are on life support medication for a transplant or severe diabetes, you MUST continue taking your medication.

Here are some statistics from the "Dr. Oz Show".

Drug companies deliberately underestimate the dangerous side effects of their drugs and most of the information that doctors receive is from the drug companies themselves. They own the data from the trials.

It has been reported that these drug companies invent new diseases to sell more of their drugs, drugs that target the symptoms not the causes of the ailment. Of course, if you don't have the disease in the first place (placebo disease), you will get better quickly and only have to deal with the side effects of the drug which may, of course, lead to your doctor prescribing additional drugs.

Fasten your seat belts for this one – the more drugs you take the greater the percentage you will experience adverse side effects.

During a 12 month period if you are taking:

2 drugs there is a 10% chance of these adverse side effects

3 drugs there is a 30% chance of   ,,   ,,   ,,   ,,

5 drugs there is a 60% chance of   ,,   ,,   ,,   ,,

7 drugs there is a 80% chance of   ,,   ,,   ,,   ,,

I believe these percentages are much higher.

Please note some drug companies boast that you can take fewer pills with their product. To this end I urge you to take note and add up the dosage of the pills. For example, if 2 pills are the same dosage as 8 pills, you are probably better off spacing the dosage out with the 8 pills rather than taking one large dose which puts a greater strain on your body. Ultimately, you should wean yourself off this medication (unless it is for life support) and follow suggestions for a natural remedy that will address the root of the problem not just the symptoms.

Adult vaccines – this is necessary if you are traveling out of the country and will be exposed to exotic diseases such as malaria, typhoid, etc., but here is what some drug companies are proposing – that you take a vaccine to a disease that is very rare in the United States and that you may very well have been vaccinated against as a child. Why??? Because they want to sell more drugs and vaccines are drugs. Not only do they want you to take their vaccines but you may be exposing yourself to a live virus of the very disease you are trying to guard against and can be transmitted to other family members in a certain time window. Now some vaccines are in killed form but you have to investigate to find out which ones are killed and which are live, the live being much more dangerous and contagious. A vague answer from your doctor probably means either he does not know or he does not want to tell you

WHAT ARE WE THINKING?

The answer to that question is that most of us are NOT thinking. We shop at the supermarkets and assume that everything in the store is safe and nutritious for us to eat. And if we have some ailment, it's okay to take any drug pertinent to our ailment whether prescribed or over the counter.

It may surprise some people that the reason persons age quickly and are susceptible to so many illnesses is that most food at the majority of super-markets is unhealthy for one reason or another. This does not apply to all the food or all supermarkets, Whole Foods Supermarket is one of the safer ones that I know of.

Antibiotics, hormones and drugs in meat and poultry are simply bad for our bodies by throwing our systems out of balance. Imbalance in our bodily systems is one of the causes of illness. When our bodies are robbing Peter to pay Paul, something has to give and it usually is our health.

Then there is the matter of chemicals sprayed on our produce whether it is fresh, canned, or frozen. You can't escape these substances unless you buy organic which isn't always available.

Let us not forget all the processed high fat snacks invite cardiac arrest. And with all that refined sugar, diabetes can happen at any time. There are at least 1 million or more Americans who have diabetes and don't know it.

Have you ever read a label that stated "artificial colors, artificial flavors? Webster defines artificial as "not by nature, not natural, made in imitation of or as a substitute for something natural, pretended". In short, they are non food ingredients blended in with real food as cheap additives, fillers, or flavoring agents. HAVE YOU EVER GONE OUT TO LUNCH DOWN AT THE LOCAL CHEMICAL PLANT? WOULD YOU PURCHASE FROM A RESTAURANT OR SUPERMARKET THAT ADVERTISED "OUR PRODUCTS AND/OR FOOD IS ONLY PART FOOD, THE REST IS HARMFUL CHEMICALS AND SUBSTANCES THAT WILL HURT YOUR BODY"? I don't think so and yet that is exactly what we are eating on a day to day basis and thinking nothing of it.

There is massive denial in our country, denial that says "if it's allowed to be in our food how bad can it be". Or "I just don't care it tastes so good, I can't stop eating it".

Let's say you have developed cancer (heaven forbid). Cancer is a disease of a weakened immune system. Some of the most common treatments for cancer are chemotherapy and radiation, both of which are serious immune depressants. If you are fortunate enough to survive these treatments, you are left in a compromised immune state which is an invitation for cancer to reoccur. This is why these patients have to be so closely monitored.

One should be aware, though, that the earlier you discover any disease that higher your chances for alternative therapy to work. Changing one's diet is an absolute must to get the body back in balance.

Again, with autoimmune diseases that are the result of the malfunction of one's immune system, immune depressing drugs are given to help with the symptoms. I recall death being listed as one of the potential side effects. This means that your immune system can become so weak that you can't defend yourself against any illness that comes your way, sometimes death being the end result.

One can readily see why these problems send health care costs spiriling upward. Most drugs are 180 degrees away from the right choice for the body. It has been reported that there actually is a shortage of many of the name brand drugs but this doesn't seem to satisfy the drug companies. They now are attempting to market drugs as a preventative for some diseases, in other words to healthy people. Children are now a main target in their sights.

And let's not forget our pets, particularly those once a month flea and tick drops that can cause seizures and death. Again, the more drugs you put in your system the more your body will become unbalanced and become susceptible to various diseases. It's planet backwards again.

The warning label on most drugs should read "WARNING: Avoid Dying".

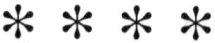

CHAPTER 23
Why Doctors Can Be Dangerous

Don't get me wrong, if you have a car accident or some form of trauma, you absolutely need medical attention. However, in the case of an illness the margin for error greatly increases because of the doctor's "textbook syndrome".

Doctors are taught in medical school that if a patient has "X" disease, then the prescribed treatment is "Y". The problem with this is that a whole list of variables does not get taken into account making DOCTORS THE NUMBER 3 CAUSE OF DEATH IN THE US following heart disease and cancer.

During the writing of this book I developed an upper respiratory inflammation. It had been a long cold winter and I was inside writing most of the time which I'm sure contributed to this ailment. Finally, I went down to the local Immediate Care facility near me to make sure that I had nothing that was life threatening.

They hooked me up to one of those finger monitors that show how well one's lungs are processing oxygen (among other things). My reading was a 92 which was low, 97-98 was the normal range . This prompted everyone to announce I needed a "breathing treatment", my first one ever. After 10 minutes breathing into this tube with medication and oxygen my lung capacity values were read and there was NO CHANGE. Another "treatment" was then ordered and I had another 10 minutes of the same treatment. This time there was a change. MY BREATHING CAPACITY VALUES HAD DECLINED 3 POINTS TO 89.

Was this not a clue to everyone that this drug not only was not working but was actually impeding my breathing? Nevertheless, I was given a prescription for this same drug to be used several times a day. We'll call this drug #1. There was another surprise in store for me with this drug. Something in its contents caused my metabolism to speed up to the point where I lost 3 1/2 lbs overnight. Now if I were to take this drug #1 for a week as prescribed, I could have conceivably lost 25 LBS IN 1 WEEK. The strain alone on my heart could have been fatal but this was what the current textbook recommendations suggested. Needless to say I did not have this prescription filled.

Drug #2 prescribed was a anti inflammatory with steroids (immune depressant). Again, this was only to treat the symptoms not cure the original cause of my breathing problem. This was to be administered by inhaler at least twice a day. I knew if the CAUSE of the inflammation were treated, my breathing would return to normal without putting immune depressants into my system. But this was not part of the textbook protocol. And yes, I did NOT have this prescription filled either.

Drug #3 was a heavy dose of antibiotics which will only help if the cause of the problem is bacterial. I presented with no temperature and my sputum was clear indicating no infection. Also, I was given a leaflet stating that the probable cause of my problem was viral and that ANTIBIOTICS WOULD BE OF NO USE IN THIS CASE. Antibiotics can and do weaken your immune system as they put a strain on the body's systems. I had already tried this drug before going to the doctor. I had some left over from a tooth abscess and it had NOT worked.

Drug #4 was an over the counter mucous remover and expectorant. After a day on this drug (the one drug I did take) I switched to another brand in a milder form as the original one completely took away my appetite depriving me of all nutrition.

All together I was told to take 10 DOSES/DAY of these various drugs at a time when I was 67 years old and not accustomed to taking drugs of any kind. Drugs can hit you much harder when you are not used to taking them – not that you should be. Also, add in the fact that I was not eating at all. Why was I given all these drugs without any other considerations? Because the textbook protocol stated that this is the method of treatment. And NONE of these doses addressed the ROOT CAUSE of the problem.

Inasmuch as I was not suicidal and have a medical background I elected to use the natural remedies for both bacterial and viral problems – remedies that would build my body up and not just treat the symptoms. Had I taken all this medication I have no doubt that I would have ended up in the hospital where they would have undoubtedly given me MORE DRUGS which could have proved fatal.

Instead I used freeze dried Echinacea Juice capsules for bacterial problems and Lomatium Isolate for viral problems both by the Eclectic Company and recovered without assaulting my body with an array of substances that would weaken me.

A sad commentary is that if you should try to explain this rationale to a doctor, most of them simply would not understand what you are talking about because they are truly brainwashed. We need more alternative medicine establishments if we are to survive this drug onslaught.

Case in point about the lack of understanding of medication – many years ago I was seeing a dentist for a type of inflammation in my mouth, As a remedy, he prescribed medication and I was instructed to take 2 tablets initially. Knowing my sensitivity to drugs and not knowing how I would react, I took only 1 tablet. I jumped in the shower shortly after taking the medication and for some reason the hot water of the shower caused a reaction with the medication. I became very dizzy, sick to my stomach and could not stand. Knowing that these symptoms would pass as the medication wore off. I just waited it out and within the hour things got better.

Here's the point! When I told the doctor/dentist what had happened, he had a total "fit" and yelled and screamed at me over the phone for taking only 1 tablet and disobeying his instructions to take 2 tablets. If I had taken 2 tablets, I might have lost consciousness, yet all he could think about was the textbook and his ego. Watch out for doctors with the "God complex".

Americans are the number 1 prescription drug users in the world and a large percentage of these drugs simply are not necessary. In addition, they are driving health care costs and premiums up substantially. It seems to be a guarded secret as to how much "monetary incentive" doctors receive based on the amount of drugs they prescribe.

In all fairness there must be some doctors who are not in this category.

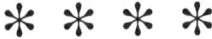

CHAPTER 24
Something All Parents Should Know

The chronological age that a child's brain is fully developed to maturity is a minimum of 21 years, possibly a little longer, specifically the frontal part of the brain that governs reason and the ability to project the consequences of their actions. Simply put, when a teenager or younger child uses recreational drugs, he/she does not realize the harmful and deadly consequences even when told and shown repeatedly.

For instance, texting while driving is very dangerous. Teens think it is perfectly safe to do this and that they have everything under control. It takes an accident in which they are responsible for them to understand, but then it's too late.

Drinking alcohol while driving, one is 5 times more likely to have an accident.

Texting while driving, one is 27 times more likely to have an accident.

Think about it—17 or 18 year olds are not allowed to vote, yet they can get behind the wheel of a moving vehicle and text while driving. Some states prohibit texting while driving, but this is very hard to enforce as they usually text in their laps out of sight.

Cell phone radiation destroys brain cells more rapidly in children under 18 more readily than that of an adult. Of course, adults are in danger also.

SAT SCORES ARE DROPPING IN HEAVILY MICROWAVED CITIES OVER THE U.S. CHILDREN ARE NOW DYING OF BRAIN CANCER.

See www.antennasearch.com and click on "Towers".

Some more statistics:

Nearly 2/3 of kids try illicit drugs before they finish high school

40% of children have tried alcohol by the time they reach 8th grade

63% have procured the alcohol from their own homes or their friend's home, Those who start at age 13 or earlier are much more likely to have an alcohol dependency later in life. KIDS WHO DRINK ALCOHOL ARE 50 TIMES MORE LIKELY TO USE COCAINE.

These statistics are likely to increase in the coming years. Statistics don't lie either. A larger percentage of fatal car accidents are proportionately higher the younger the driver is. Teens have the largest percentage of these accidents. The immature brain just doesn't "get it".

Likewise, a high level of fatalities occur in the military with soldiers in their teens or early 20's. WHY IS ONE ALLOWED TO ELIST IN THE MILITARY WITH A MUCH GREATER CHANCE OF GETTING KILLED WHEN ONE'S BRAIN IS NOT FULLY DEVELOPED? The responsible thing to do would be to change the military enrollment age to 21 as well as the voting age.. However, enrollments could very well decrease because at an older age one might think twice about the consequences of their actions.

Crime is another example of this lack of brain development. Teens can commit crimes and the thought that they may die or go to prison has no meaning to them. As parents you need to keep a closer eye on your children because they are not mentally "there" yet. So many parents have been fooled just because they thought "my son/daughter is very mature for his/her age". "My child would NEVER do drugs".

A common mistake a large number of parents make is trying to be their child's friend. Meanwhile, Sally or Johnny is surfing the internet where drug use is routinely glorified along with instructions on how to make or procure these drugs. The only way to keep a tight rein on your children is to be, in part, their parole officer. It is far better to have them resent you a little than to have them end up in a rehab facility or prison which may or may not work. You may have to keep track of them by noticing whether or not their pupils dilate and contract normally and have them submit to random drug tests with severe penalties if they fail. Some tests are available at most local pharmacies without a prescription. Denial is the worst possible thing you can do.

Hopefully by the time they are 18 they will be on the right path to completely recognizing right from wrong, but they must be given specific examples of the right path on a regular basis along with some discipline. At some point in time most teenagers will probably hate their parents. It's part of the hormonal changes. Most of the time they will outgrow these mood swings. Studies have shown that deep down most teens like being disciplined because it shows them that their parents care. By discipline I mean taking away privileges and sticking to it. Harsh physical correction should be avoided.

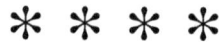

CHAPTER 25
The Invisible Price Tag

Let me explain. Our bodies are designed to breathe a certain quality air and eat a certain type and quality of food with built in mechanisms to get rid of toxic elements (within reason). But our lifestyles, for the most part, have thrown caution and reason to the wind. We just assume everything will be all right and, if not, there are always the doctors with their medications and/or surgeries.

Every time we deviate from the path that our bodies were designed for there is a price to pay. Drugs, for example, put a major strain on our bodies with their multitude of side effects.

Warning: If you are on a life support drug such as an immune depressant because of a transplant or any other drug that is necessary to keep you alive, you must continue to stay on your medication.

The wrong foods are another example of the invisible price tag. The vast array of altered foods with added chemicals, hormones, drugs and refining can cause internal problems in our systems which are not readily apparent. But, like a ticking time bomb, illness and disease arrives at a later date because of the imbalance and clogging of our systems. It's a cause and effect. If you ingest carcinogens, you greatly increase your odds of contracting cancer. Nitrates and nitrites in bacon and most cold cuts are a good example of carcinogens. I say "most" because companies such as Applegate Farms have actually had the foresight to remove these harmful substances from their bacon, cold cuts, etc. Halleluiah!

Refined foods with all their nutrients stripped away through processing enter the body in an imperfect state. This causes the body to search within itself to make up the deficiencies in enzymes and missing ingredients to be able to process and digest this food. This leaves our internal body's bank accounts in a state of depletion and eventually exhausted. At this point illness and disease are a sure thing.

Wouldn't it be much simpler just to give one's body what it requires in the first place? Yet, at this point in time it will require some effort until the food manufacturers and preparers get on board. Fast junk food ought to be labeled "faster death". Other chapters in this book will aid you in this cause.

This really is the way to minimize your heath care costs!!

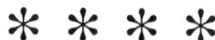

CHAPTER 26
The Causes And Effects Of
Spinal Misalignments

C- cervical (neck)   T- thoracic (back)   L- Lumbar (upper hip)

S – sacrum (lower hip)

Spinal vertebrae and discs being out of alignment may cause irritation to the nervous system and affect the structures, organs and functions of one's body as listed below:

C1 – Blood supply to the head, pituitary gland, scalp, bones of the face, brain, inner and middle ear, parasympathetic nervous system

Malfunctions – Headaches, nervousness, insomnia, head colds, high blood pressure, migraine headaches, nervous breakdown, amnesia, chronic tiredness, dizziness

C2 –Eyes optic nerves, auditory nerves, sinuses, mastoid bones, tongue, forehead

Malfunctions –Sinus trouble, allergies, crossed eyes, deafness, eye trouble earache, fainting spells, certain causes of blindness

C3 – Cheeks, outer ear, face bones, teeth, trigeminal nucleus

Malfunctions –Neuralgia, neuritis, acne or pimples, eczema

C4 – Nose, lips, mouth, eustachian tube, tonsils

Malfunctions – Hay fever catarrh, hearing loss, adenoids, tonsillitis

C5 – Vocal chords, neck glands, pharynx, shoulders, thyroid gland

Malfunctions – Laryngitis, hoarseness, sore throat, pain in the upper arm/ shoulder, thyroid conditions

C6 – Neck, muscles, elbows

Malfunctions – Stiff neck, whooping cough, croup, tennis elbow, colds

C7 – Arms from the elbows down, including hands, wrists, fingers

Malfunctions – Pain in lower arms and hands

T1 – Esophagus, trachea

Malfunctions – Asthma, cough, difficulty breathing, shortness of breath

T2 - Heart, including valves, coronary arteries and bronchioles

Malfunctions – functional heart and chest conditions, asthma, high/low blood pressure

T3 – Lungs, bronchial tubes

Malfunctions – bronchitis, pleurisy, pneumonia, congestion, influenza, asthma

T4 – Gall bladder, common bile duct

Malfunctions – gall bladder conditions, jaundice, shingles

T5 – Liver, solar plexus, blood

Malfunctions –liver conditions, fevers, anemia, poor circulation

T6 – Stomach

Malfunctions – stomach troubles, including nervous stomach, indigestion, heartburn, dyspepsia, ulcers

T7 – Pancreas, duodenum

Malfunctions – ulcers, gastritis, blood sugar levels

T8 – Spleen

Malfunction – lowered resistance

T9 – Adrenal and supra-renal glands

Malfunctions – allergies, hives, energy level

T10 – Kidneys

Malfunctions – kidney troubles, hardening of the arteries, chronic tiredness, nephritis, pyelitis

T11 – Kidneys, ureters

Malfunctions – skin conditions such as acne, pimples, eczema or boils

T12 – Small intestines, lymph circulations

Malfunctions – rheumatism, pimples, certain types of sterility

1L – Large intestine, inguinal rings

Malfunctions – constipation, colitis, dysentery, diarrhea, some ruptures of hernias

2L – Appendix, abdomen, upper leg

Malfunctions – cramps, appendicitis, thigh pain

3L - Sex organs, uterus, bladder, knees

Malfunctions – bladder troubles, menstrual troubles, such as painful or irregular periods, miscarriages, bed wetting, impotency, change of life symptoms, many knee pains

4L – Prostate gland, muscles of the lower back, sciatic nerve

Malfunctions – sciatica, lumbago, difficult, painful, or too frequent urination, backaches

5L - Lower legs, ankles, feet, sciatic nerve

Malfunctions – poor circulation in the legs, swollen ankles, weak ankles and arches, cold feet, weakness in the legs, leg cramps, sciatica, varicose veins

Sacrum – Hip bones, buttocks, groin

Malfunctions – sacro-iliac conditions, spinal curvatures, groin pain

Coccyx (tailbone) – rectum, anus

Malfunctions – hemorrhoids (piles), pruritis (itching), pain at the end of the spine upon sitting

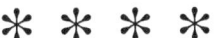

CHAPTER 27
Harmful Electromagnetic Fields

Electromagnetic fields are all around us, everywhere we go, and they produce a certain amount of harm to our bodies. Once again, denial is the prevailing emotion with reference to the electromagnetic field radiation from our cell phones, computers, fluorescent lighting, etc. Since we can't see these fields, we act as though they don't exist.

EMF's have been linked to Alzheimers, breast cancer, depression, heart disease, allergies, autism, headaches, hormone changes, premature births, low birth weights, immune system damage, nerve damage, sleep disturbances, cataracts, and sperm abnormalities.

Also, there have been reports of eye irritation and cataracts from high levels of radio frequency and microwave radiation.

Our bodies, which are electric in nature, respond favorably to negative ions such as those produced by waves crashing on the beach. Conversely, cell phones, computers, etc. give off positive ions which are very harmful to the body. The wrong type of 'current' can have negative effects, such as brain cancer. The cell phone frequencies can alter DNA replication and it is these cells that can become cancerous. A study with rats showed an aggressive growth in leukemia cells after exposure to these fields.

No one is asking you to give up your electronic equipment, but we're supposed to be intelligent human beings. There are several products available which help with the effects of the EMF's. The cost is minor compared to the major damage being done to us from these fields.

I personally use the Q-link SRT3 pendant. This pendant balances and clarifies one's energies and is proven to reduce the effects of stress on one's mind and body, allowing one to experience enhanced well-being, increased performance and improved quality of life. This pendant has been shown to help reduce the negative effects of EMFS generated by electronic equipment.

This also is very helpful for 'jet lag' and pro golfers swear it helps their golf game. There are many other products on the market that claim to help the body withstand EMF's and can be researched on line.

There are many other products along this line now available.

CELL TOWERS – are springing up all over the place and their radiation poses some severe health threats if one lives too close to them. There is a web site www.antennasearch.com whereby you can type in your address and zip code and click on the towers and antennas link and a map will pop up and show you exactly where they are in relation to your address along with a scale of miles. The map uses 4 a mile radius as a safety net and I wasn't pleased with the 24 towers that came up near my address.

The main concern with this radiation is that it causes a lack of quantity and quality sleep which leads to all sorts of diseases for millions of people, some even leading to death.

Brace yourself, but that Bluetooth around your ear has been linked to hearing loss and brain cancer with at least one pending lawsuit.

POWER LINES – living or being near power lines is a real "no no". I once was house hunting where the development had power lines running straight through the center. I purchased a gauss meter to determine the length in feet when the EMF was no longer dangerous. The result was 1200 feet away from the tower when the red light on the meter went "off", I didn't purchase in the development because the power lines were just too close.

Living with power lines on or near your property can be very dangerous to your health. And, oh yes, the builders are able to purchase this land at a substantial discount. The utility companies may tell everyone that there are no harmful effects, but the gauss meter doesn't lie.

Please see chapter on Explicit Dangers Of Microwaves and the chapter on Something All Parents Should Know for the dangers to children from cell phone radiation.

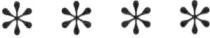

CHAPTER 28
Indoor Pollution

There is an invisible health problem lurking in most homes, one that you would never suspect. Now before I reveal this villain, please keep in mind that action is required on your part to change the things in your life that are undermining your health. Just because you've been living a certain way all your life does not mean it's the right way. Just look at the medical bills this country incurs.

Okay, here goes. Please read the whole story before throwing the book down. Non vented natural gas appliances give off an enormous source of indoor pollution. Primarily, the combustion is incomplete, meaning that it does not completely burn, leaving the non combusted particles to get into your body through your lungs. The incomplete combustion contains methane which is an asphyxiant, which has suffocation properties.

This should be of special interest to people with asthma, allergies, respiratory problems, chemical sensitivity or any other breathing problem. Heated natural gas creates nitrogen dioxide, carbon monoxide, hydrocarbons, formaldehyde, etc. which sticks to your food so that you eat these chemicals as well as inhale them. These substances can sensitize you to other substances in the environment making you allergic to things you normally would not react to. Non vented fireplace stoves just pour this pollution into your home.

Also, gas combustion produces water vapor which contributes to molds, bacteria, viruses, dust mites, etc. It sticks to your clothes with gas dryers which should have more than a side vent which is not adequate. I have heard that gas clothes dryers have a tendency to make your clothes yellow.

Wood burning fireplace smoke has a whole host of deadly pollutants. These pollutants go up the chimney and then pollute the neighborhood.

New carpet should be aired out for at least 3 days before being placed in the living environment because of all the chemicals in its manufacture.

Indoor ionizers should be purchased very carefully as the ones that produce ozone have a harmful effect on one's lungs.

Also, it is prudent not to live on a busy street where there is constant vehicle traffic as the carbon monoxide that the cars and trucks give off enters your home (our homes are not air tight) and causes a whole host of problems.

Summary – electric cooking, in my opinion, is the safest followed by induction cooking. Some worthwhile advantages would be your children can't set fire to themselves and their clothing as well as having an electronic lock that only older children would be able to operate.

Switching to natural cleaners such as the Biokleen product line can have a significant impact on reducing indoor pollution. This particular line of products really works.

Induction cooking produces "electromagnetic radiation" and the jury is still out on this. Persons with pacemakers or any other type of implanted devices might want to exercise more caution with reference to induction cooking.

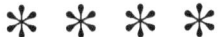

PSYCHOLOGICAL STRESS FACTORS

CHAPTER 29
The Disease Of Denial
(Are you in harms way?)

Probably the majority of the U.S. population is in some form of denial. This is dangerous because it not only leaves you unprepared, but prevents you from taking the proper steps to protect yourself.

Of course, one of the main issues is one's health. If you are 30 lbs or more overweight and are ignoring those pounds, you're in denial. These overweight pounds tend to increase without much effort on your part because denial is keeping you from taking control of your weight and your health. And when disease hits you, you can blame it on heredity or your friend or relative who keeps bringing you the junk food. It's time to take control of your situation. "Just say no" doesn't only apply to drugs. This means saying "no" to your children and "no" to the junk food on the supermarket shelves when it 'accidentally' drops into your shopping cart. Not bringing the disease makers (improper food) into your home is ¾ of the battle.

The fact that we cannot trace most diseases directly back to a poor lifestyle allows us to blame something or someone else.

Children are especially hurt by not being trained to eat the right foods. Try a daily visit to a weight scale, preferable in the am without clothes before eating. This way your weight can't get out of control. If it starts to increase, take steps to exercise more, cut calories or eat more sensibly.

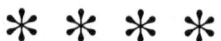

CHAPTER 30
Relieving Stress By
Being Prepared

By this I don't mean running for the tranquilizer bottle or leaving for Tahiti. A great deal of hidden stress can be vanquished by having "back up" supplies of food and water, a solar generator that does not require gasoline to run, a back up bank account and whatever else you feel would be helpful to have a surplus supply of.

A personal example would be my back up supply of cat food. At one time the store where I purchase this food was very erratic with its' deliveries – I had no idea how much stress this was putting on me until I decided to store a few weeks of extra cat food. When the cat food delivery to the store was postponed, I didn't have to scramble trying to figure out where I could buy this specialized product.

Look into any programs your local utility has with reference to solar panels. Here in New Jersey they offer a huge rebate with the balance being paid off with a loan. If you have enough solar panels, the electric company PAYS you each month, therefore, in addition to not having an electric bill, you can put the money you would have spent on the bill plus any rebates toward paying off the loan which is usually 5 years. You will be saving lots of money and have peace of mind that you'll be protected during a power failure.

The following suggestion is easier said than done, but in the long run you probably will wish you had done it sooner. You need to be truthful with yourself and identify the people and things in your life that are systematically draining you. You need to say "no" to these people and things. Most important, stop giving yourself permission to experience stress by associating with them. Avoid them, their phone calls and, if necessary, their friends. Feeling guilty almost always means you're on the wrong track.

This chapter is not for those of you who prefer to be oblivious to our intensifying weather patterns. The millions, if not billions, of tons of carbon monoxide we dump into the atmosphere, is starting to have a major effect on our weather especially in the form of heavy rain and drought. As a scientist, I can tell you that I am absolutely convinced the weather patterns are going to get much worse within 5 years or less. A while back I heard a rather startling statistic. If we were able to stop ALL harmful emissions into the atmosphere, the CO_2 levels would continue to rise and not level out for 30 YEARS. And here we are increasing our emissions. The dire consequences of this increase still remain to be seen.

A while ago in an effort to downsize my home I was exploring a smaller housing development on line when to my surprise, I found that the development was 5 blocks away from a major river. To make matters even worse the river turned so that the river was also 5 blocks from the side of the development as well as the front. In my opinion, this is a disaster waiting to happen. To those of you who live on a flood plain I would respectively suggest you move if at all possible. Now I'm not suggesting we build an ark, just be practical with a large helping of common sense.

The next time you have a power failure try to take note of how uncomfortable you feel, especially if it lasts for several hours. Don't you breathe a deep sign of relief when the power is restored? I know I do. Pretend the power is not going to come on for days or weeks and act accordingly by being more prepared. Yes, this is expensive but our electrical grid system in this country is getting older and is very antiquated. Having a solar source of power is one of the smartest things that one can do. Most of us are not prepared for a gasoline shortage which will affect food deliveries and almost everything else you can imagine. A generator powered by gas could become useless in the event of a gasoline interruption.

Having a greenhouse would be for the serious person who wants to be prepared.

And, of course, the ultimate preparation would be to have your body prepared for any onslaught of disease by taking the precaution of eliminating all poisons and altered foods from your diet, drinking water and a non ozone air purifier with at least one charcoal filter.

RELIEVING STRESS IN GENERAL

We all hear of the many tragedies in this world and most of us have personally experienced our share. We sincerely hope no more misfortune befalls us, but we seem powerless to the winds of fate. This produces an underlying stress on our systems which we may not realize exists. Stress encourages the body to produce more energy in the form of fatty acids and glucose which requires the liver to produce and secrete more LDL cholesterol.

There are precautions we can take for reducing hidden stress, stress we may not even be aware of. My way of dealing with this hidden stress may sound a little neurotic, but it works for me. I call it preparing for the 'worst case scenario"

Most of it is just plain safety.. Before you leave the house for any reason, even if it's just going to the corner store, make sure ALL your appliances are off and any hazard that could start a fire has been taken care of. Case in point, I recently received a recall on my dishwasher to replace a part in the control panel that had been causing fires in people's homes. But with my 'shut off all appliances policy before leaving the house', this would never have happened to me.

Also make sure you lock your doors and your windows with the exception if you have pets that need ventilation. If the weatherman says it is going to be 75 degrees, plan for 85 degrees just to be safe.

Sign up for a link to your cell phone from your power company to alert you to a power failure. Dogs, cats and other pets can suffer from heat stroke if it gets too hot. Leave the basement door open (if you have a basement), but first remove any hazards that could injure your pets. Leaving the basement door open is not necessary in winter. Remember, after the fact is too late.

Now you're ready for the road. I like to pretend that ALL the other drivers on the road have just escaped from an insane asylum which is not too far from the truth. This makes me drive very defensively and allow a couple of extra car lengths from the car in front in case some nut decides to brake at the last moment.

If you are out alone at night, carry pepper spray on your key chain and learn self defense from a quick training course. When entering your car, hit your car's lock button FIRST before you do anything else, even before you put your key in the ignition or fasten your seat belt. If someone approaches your car to open your car door, you can start the engine and take off. If the perpetrator has a knife and your windows are closed, your can still get away. If there's a gun involved, you may have to surrender your belongings and vehicle, but only you can make that call at the time. Just don't put yourself in a position where you are alone at night in a dark parking lot or garage or street. Have someone accompany you, preferably a man. Don't assume you are safe. And, please, don't go jogging alone, especially in the woods.

With regard to taking supplements for relieving stress, I would recommend a whole food multivitamin and extra B Complex by Mega Food, as well as an adrenal glandular.

By being aware of what is really going on out in one's environment we can take the proper precautions. This 'preparing for the worst' method allows you to be prepared in advance for almost anything.

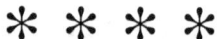

CHAPTER 31
Never Assume – Ever

With each passing decade of age one cannot help but accumulate wisdom from life's experiences. One of the most important, if not THE most important, is training yourself not to assume facts without all the pertinent information.

Case in point – I recently called the electric company to verify my balance as I was going to pay my pill. The girl on the phone gave me an amount that was $20 less than the amount on my statement. I told her I wanted to pay the larger amount just to be sure my bill was not $20 past due. "Big deal" you might say, however, I had signed up with an alternate electric supplier whose rate was less and if my account had gone past due, I would have defaulted back to the original supplier with the higher price.

Subsequently, a call back to verify that my payment had gone through revealed that there was no such thing as the $20 difference in my favor. Had I assumed that the original girl was correct it would have cost me financially.

With my next bill I discovered that when they replaced my defective electric meter, someone added 1100 kilowatts from the old meter to the reading on the new meter. This represented more that $160. Good thing I did not assume the bill was correct.

Another case in point – After switching telephone servers I discovered that I had forgotten to block my caller ID that displays my phone number to the person I have called. A call to the phone company took care of this but when I inquire4 if I could unblock my number by hitting "*82" they told me their system was not set up that way, that I would have to go into a particular website and disable the feature and then enable it after my phone call.

This did not sound correct so I tried unblocking with the "*82" and it worked. The moral here is that you just can't assume the person at the other end of the line knows what they are talking about.

A story of peaches – while shopping at a local summer farm market I noticed that the peaches were marked $4.99 for 2 quarts and $7.99 for 4 quarts, a supposed saving of $1.99. One day I decided to weigh both these items as the 4 quart bag just did not look twice the size of the 2 quart one. Normally one would assume that these prices reflected double the weight but the scale proved differently. The bag weighed only 5 lbs instead of 6.

Never assume the computer in a store knows what's on sale. I've seen this happen in supermarkets and more recently in an electronics store. I was purchasing a wireless mouse for my computer that was on sale for around half the price, however, the computer scanned it at full price. When I protested, both the manager and the sales person told me that it was a different model that was on sale, not the one I had selected. I almost believed them, but something told me to go to the shelf and check. Sure enough, the computer was wrong, the manager was wrong and the sales person was WRONG. They had to credit me and charge the sale price. That $20 is much better off in my wallet than their register.

There are so many instances in life where we automatically assume something is true when, in reality, it is not. It's simply a matter of training yourself to question and verify things that are told you as well as things you observe.

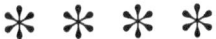

CHAPTER 32
Those Who Will Not Forgive

Probably most of us know someone who fits into this category. As an example, some years ago I ran into someone I knew who happened to mention to me that I needed to start wearing my seat belt. When I told her that I started wearing my seat belt constantly after the law took effect which was 2 years prior to our immediate conversation, she started berating me and telling me that I was a bad person for not wearing my seat belt. Even after I told her that I now liked wearing it, she couldn't see the change. It wasn't as though I had had an accident or caused someone bodily harm, it was just that she wasn't about to give up her vendetta on the subject. At that point there was no conversation, just my hasty exit.

Then there are the persons who enjoy believing the worst about anyone. Maybe it makes them feel superior and perhaps satisfies their jealousy. This type of person will continue to believe a lie about you even if there is overwhelming proof to the contrary.

The reason this is being mentioned here is that these people can have a major impact on your health which can result in additional medical bills. Please take note that the majority of these people will not change. Some might with counseling and discovering what the root of their problem is. The best solution is not to have anything to do with them.

I know a man who was very attached to his mother and when she died in her late sixties (way too young), he channeled his grief by blaming his sister for her death. The mother's diet and lifestyle were not optimum and she contracted cancer. How this could possibly be the fault of his sister is certainly illogical. Some people just need to have a scapegoat. Interestingly enough, his diet could use some major improvement especially as he is now approaching the age at which his mother died. This type of emotional poison directs inward and can shorten one's life expectancy.

After countless attempts over the years to win her brother's friendship, the sister finally realized that it was in her best health interest to disassociate herself from him. If you have a relative, friend or acquaintance that fits this category, it just isn't worth the toll it takes on your body, even if you can't see it.

Habitual liars are another category of people to avoid. The first category is the 'people pleaser' who will tell you what he/she thinks you want to hear and will put him/her in a favorable light. The next category is the person who lies repeatedly to cover his tracks even if his actions are lawful. This type of person lies so repeatedly that I wonder if he/she can distinguish fact from fiction.

There are more categories than this, but I think you get the idea. These are people to avoid because the invisible and visible stress they place on you is damaging to your health. The more stress we avoid the healthier we will be.

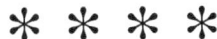

CHAPTER 33
False Or Sneaky Advertising

False advertising is everywhere. Manufacturers seem to be able to say almost anything they want short of their product curing disease.

Lower calorie claim – one product will claim to have fewer calories which it actually does, but the product may be the 6 oz. size instead of an 8 oz. size which is 25% less product or 25% fewer calories. They haven't lied, they just haven't told the whole truth.

Food commercials tell you how healthy their product is, but a good deal of the time it's a distortion of the truth. The latest is "whole grain". If you read the actual product ingredients, you will find that the actual amount of whole grain can be just a fraction of the total grain in the product.

A certain cereal manufacturer advertises multigrain flakes with honey on their cereal box. A closer inspection of the ingredients reveals that at least one grain is not a whole grain, that there is refined sugar which is much higher up on the ingredient list than the honey, BHT preservative (a total "no no") and what appears to be a whole medley of synthetic vitamins.

Investigate foods that claim to have "no preservatives" or "no trans fat", etc. They eliminate one unhealthy ingredient but don't tell you about the other unhealthy ingredients that remain such as refined white flour, sugar, etc.

One of my favorite advertisements is the mascara commercial, not all of them but one in particular ad shows the 'after' shot with the model wearing false eyelashes.

Here on the East Coast we now have the choice to select which natural gas and/or electric supplier we wish to buy from. Usually the one with the best rate prevails. However, you need to compare the ACTUAL rates of your current utility supplier because the rate the competitors list in their brochure for your current provider usually is higher than it really is. This makes their rate look more appealing. I recently switched my electric supplier to save the 20% they advertised. It turned out that I am only saving 10% and when my first supplier has a rate change for the winter, the original provider may be slightly less expensive. Fortunately, I made sure the current company has no cancellation fee as some do. If you lock in for a year and your old company lowers their rates, you are stuck paying the higher rate for the period of time on your contract. Also, these promotional rates have a time limit and you will undoubtedly pay more when the promo rate expires.

Then there's the very unbelievably inexpensive cell phone monthly rates. The catch is that everything is extra, every minute you talk, every option, etc. which can make this plan more expensive than one that gives you a free number of minutes each month.

It's amazing to what lengths some companies will go to lure you to their product and/or services. Recently I opened a money mailer to find that a particular company was advertising to clean the vents and trunk lines of one's home for $35, a service which normally costs hundreds of dollars. It turned out that there is a consultation fee of $65, each vent is $9 for sanitizing (most homes have at least 11-15 vents) and every time a trunk line turns a corner it is another $65. The girl answering the phone actually told me that most homes cost from $300-$1000 not $35 as advertised. Heaven knows what other costs they add on.

The problem with a lot of today's advertising (not all) is the sin of omission. The advertisers deliberately don't tell you what the product or premium is really going to cost you over the long term.

Don't be afraid to do the math:

$50/month = $600/year or $1200 for 2 years

$300/month = $3600/year or $7200 for 2 years, etc.

Is your item really going to cost that amount of money in repairs over that time period. You probably would be better off setting up a separate savings account and pay your premium directly to the bank account each month. This will require some discipline, but the rewards will be substantial.

Also, the money could be used for a genuine emergency if need be, money that would be in someone else's pocket and gone forever.

✳ ✳ ✳ ✳

MISCELLANEOUS

CHAPTER 34
Let's Talk Health Insurance

Imagine a world where health insurance is not affordable to most people. We need to be prepared for the worst and not take our health insurance for granted.

Years ago I discovered I had a tooth abscess which required a root canal procedure to rid the infection as it was near the tip of the tooth root. At the time I was living on a meager social security check with no funds to pay for this procedure and no dental insurance. Even though I was scheduled to receive some money in a few months, no dentist would treat me. One dentist did tell me that since it was an upper abscess there was a danger the infection would migrate to the brain and that I needed to have the tooth treated immediately. Then he promptly showed me the door.

It was very disturbing to learn that my life was not worth one hour of someone's time and after all, the dentist would be paid, just not right away. Fortunately, I had Medicare insurance for the prescription which was $246.00 - my cost was $6.30. The insurance company was quick to notify me that my renewal of this drug would be limited even though I had not had a prescription filled in years.

The point here is that this was a taste of needing medical assistance with no one willing to help. I can't help but wonder what life will be like in the not too distant future as government spending currently seems to have no reins. Sooner, rather than later, health insurance WILL BECOME UNAFFORDABLE except for the very rich.

The time to take action is now and apply the contents of this book to your lifestyle. A few simple changes to one's eating habits will ward off considerable illness and disease. Unnecessary prescriptions and over the counter drugs just weaken your body while the natural remedies strengthen you. Just some simple education and application to this end is needed.

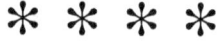

CHAPTER 35
Saving Money

There's a lot to be said about saving money and using coupons. I'm all for this but be warned that most of the food coupons I've seen are for food that is of very low quality and aren't worth the paper they're printed on. However, coupons for paper products, paper towels, toilet tissue, garbage bags, etc. are very worthwhile. Most people I know don't care what is in the food as long as they can buy it cheap. For some people there is such an inner satisfaction of putting one over on the food manufacturers that health and reasoning seem to go out the window. Ultimately, you pay 1000+ times more than you save on doctor and medical bills. You just don't see it coming.

You can call the manufacturers of wholesome foods you like and request their coupons on the various products. A number of them will be happy to comply. These coupons are usually for $1 or more and may not be subject to double couponing. When you do find a favorite item on sale, the smart thing to do is to buy several of the particular items if you can.

Do you look to the left of the shelf price of the item you are going to buy to see how the price per unit or lb. differs from the size of the box or package? The larger package is not always the best buy. Sometimes there is a much larger saving with the smaller size especially if it's on sale. Try this out with garbage bags – there can be quite a variation.

On the other hand most supermarkets have a "family pack" meat section where you can save $1 or more per lb. However, sometimes a sale on chicken, for example, will be much lower per lb. than the family pack price. Remember to purchase chickens that are raised without hormones or antibiotics.

Next tip – buy the real deal. You can pay a premium for food that has been cooked and frozen for you. Now while this may be okay once in a while, keep in mind that it takes about the same time to bake fresh chicken cutlets as it does the frozen ones (give or take a minute or two). The fresh food is so much better for you and is usually less expensive. And while your meat is baking in the oven you can throw some fresh vegetables in a stainless steel (not aluminum) steamer. A bunch of broccoli can go a long way and if your family is very small, you can cook a part of the bunch and save the rest for fresh cooking in a day or two. Please see chapter on "Harmful Effects Of Microwaves".

A real potential money saver is to higher skilled workman at the "time and materials" price rather than the "contract" price. This way you pay for only the time worked and the materials they use. The "contract" price has to factor in any unknown pitfalls or delays to the contractors and you can be sure they are coming out ahead financially.

At least 20 years ago when 401 retirement funds were "in" I did not participate. There was absolutely no logic to having strangers have access to my money, people I knew nothing about. It turned out I was correct, people have lost a great deal, if not all, of their savings to these retirement accounts. I am a strong advocate of precious metals, gold, silver and platinum as the only safe way to invest.

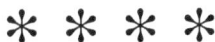

CHAPTER 36
Did You Know?

Too much vitamin C can cause a calcium deficiency and can chelate calcium out of the body.

High phosphorus intake such as in soft drinks and meat increases the need for calcium.

The effects of microgravity such as traveling in space drastically weakens one's bone structure and causes premature osteoporosis. Until scientists solve this problem a longer trip to outer space would be a death sentence.

Calcium requires magnesium, enzymes, and B6 to be incorporated into building bone. When these cocatalysts are not present in sufficient quantities, the calcium is likely to manifest as calcification of the joints, leading to tendonitis, bursitis, arthritis, and bone spurs.

The more toxic your body is the stronger the taste will be in your mouth upon awakening. You can actually get to the point where you have no "morning mouth".

Fruits and vegetables imported from other countries can, and usually do contain harmful chemicals that are banned her in the United States. This is because their laws are not as strict as ours. Be especially careful in the winter.

The day that hospital fatalities are the highest is the first Wednesday in August. This is the day the new interns from medical school begin their residency at the various hospitals (Manswers TV show).

Cooking with Teflon cookware gives off small particles that can kill your pet bird(s) when inhaled. The study did not give the cumulative effect on the lungs of humans but it can't be good. I would be wary of all non stick cookware. Please see chapter on Ailments And Diseases.

A certain flame retardant in sofa and chair cushions has been linked to cancer. Wall Street Journal Article discovery by Dr. Heather Stapleton Washington Toxins Coalition, Environmental Science and Technology Journal.

Alpha-lipoic acid (ALA) fights liver and heart disease, cancer and diabetes. In Europe a doctors was able to regenerate the livers of virtually all his patients with ALA.

Vitamin D studies have shown this vitamin to be helpful with bone health, metabolic health, cardiovascular health while promoting healthy immune cell activation. It also acts as a regulator of gene expression promoting healthy immune cell activation and cell metabolism.

Elevated blood sugar levels significantly increase your risk of heart disease and pancreatic cancer.

High blood sugar levels can affect your ability to remember and cause permanent memory loss.

Your blood sugar levels generally increase as you age, when you gain weight around your midsection, and when you eat a diet high in saturated fat.

35 minutes on your cell phone can cause your body temperature to rise as well as your blood pressure.

2% milk is very high in fat.

A patient in a hospital with high blood pressure and diabetes was given a diet high in sugar and salt. When he objected, the nurse stated that they would simply increase his blood pressure and insulin medication. Insane!

When your breath smells like fish = liver problems, urine = kidney problems, fruity = pancreas (diabetes) problems.

Enzymes boost metabolism and detoxify body.

Zinc helps to curb appetite (don't overdo).

Estrogen holds on to fat in the body.

Talcum enters via the lungs and skin and has been linked to severe physical problems.

Synthetic clothing such as polyester have a negative effect on the body as they do not allow the skin to breathe properly. 100% cotton is the best but takes some effort to find as the synthetic material usually is much cheaper. Silk and wool would be considered natural fibers.

A person with blood type "O" can find it extremely difficult to become a vegetarian. This has something to do with one's ancestry possibly centuries ago.

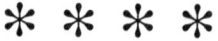

CHAPTER 37
Save Our Pets

As bad as the food available to humans can be, it is much worse for our dogs, cats, small animals, etc. Apparently animals are considered as part of a low life form therefore it does not matter if their food is sub par. Nothing could be farther than the truth. By feeding my animals the best quality food I find my vet bills are at an absolute minimum.

One of the main side effects of poor quality food is kidney failure. You take your animal to the vet and are given drugs which cause an additional strain on your pet's liver and kidneys. Some vets tell you there is simply nothing they can do and they are correct. However, there is something you can do.

If drugs and hormones in our food are bad for people, it is just as bad for our pets. One of the best quality pet foods for dogs and cats is Pet Guard which is usually sold at health food stores, not like some of the garbage that is sold at pet stores. To the best of my knowledge there are no antibiotics and/or hormones in Pet Guard. New Jersey pet stores are now starting to carry some higher quality selections. For the time being I have not seen Pet Guard on their shelves. It costs a little more but the money saved in vet bills would probably pay for the food outright.

Getting back to kidney failure I would suggest a kidney glandular given twice a day (1/3 to ½ capsule depending upon the size of your pet). Also, it is very important to feed your pet ONLY WET FOOD. Dry food takes a lot of water to process and ailing kidneys need a lot of water. Pet Guard comes in both wet and dry for dogs and cats

Next on the health list is pure water for your pets. If you won't drink tap water yourself, why is it okay to give it to your pet? The chapter in this book on Water gives a complete overview on the do's and don'ts.

Good news for cat parents. At last there is an almost dust free cat litter. This dust in most other cat litter coats everything from the TV to taking the finish off your hardwood floors. The labels say 99% dust free – not true for most brands, but Dr. Elsey's has an extensive line of cat litters and products sold at Petsmart. My cats absolutely prefer it.

The 40 lb bag of Ultra Precious Cat is the most economical but the smaller bags have a coupon book, at least at this time. It beats the name brands hands down and stays cleaner so that kitty will not be tempted to use another place. Will be updating this recommendation in my book "Alternative Health Remedies For Cats".

Alternative Health Remedies For Dogs will be coming out in 2013.

Finally, AVOID ANY PET FOOD THAT CONTAINS BY-PRODUCTS. It is my understanding that by-products legally can contain sawdust, hair, and a variety of non edible substances which will lead to illness. Ever notice how busy your vet is?

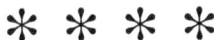

CONCLUSION

CHAPTER 38
We Need Change

As hard as this may be to believe MOST of the food available at super-markets and food stores has been refined and altered with chemicals, preservatives, additives, and/or hormones or drugs added to the point where the food is truly unhealthy for the human body. Just as you can probably run a car on kerosene or some other imitation for a while, ultimately the car will break down and wear out before its time. In other words, the aging process of the motor will be speeded up causing the motor to need replacement.

Does this sound familiar? It has to be a billion $ industry on replacement parts and transplants for the human body. Baring some genetic defect, the remainder of these needed replacements are a direct result of the abuse of one's body occurring from ignorance or an immortality complex (it will happen to the other guy, not to me).

So why do we get sick? Most of our food is being polluted and refined with additives, preservatives, hormones, drugs and chemicals to the point where it is not compatible with the human body. Our water has a gazillion harmful substances in it, (well water is still polluted with acid rain, etc), Most of the air we breathe is high in carbon monoxide and other chemicals. This puts a tremendous amount of stress and strain on our bodies. Add to this a society that is hooked on prescription drugs to say nothing of the recreational ones. It's a miracle we live as long as we do.

Until food manufacturers learn that healthy food ultimately will be their best sellers, one has to diligently read labels, shop at health food stores for foods that are in their natural state, while at the same time paying attention to your overall health picture.

THE GOAL IS TO TAKE CONTROL OF ONE'S BODY AND NOT SIT ON THE HIGHWAY OF ILLNESS AND DISEASE AND WAIT TO BE RUN OVER. This prevention method really works.

As stated earlier, I don't have a regular doctor. Disease is prevented from gaining a foothold on me because it has no place to land. Healthy tissue is naturally resistance to disease. It's only when the body gets out of balance that illness and disease find a home.

And for those nasty genetic genes that rear their ugly heads no matter what – consider this solution. If a pregnant woman is eating this refined, tainted food, it is like a checkered flag for the genes in her body to distort. And since most families tend to have the same eating habits, it may not be caused by a defective gene at all, just the wrong foods in the wrong amounts.

Here you have the recipe for success or disaster – you need to follow your own body's rules not yours!

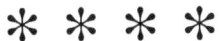

Reference Guide

This guide applies only to chapters where specific references to products are mentioned.

Chapter 2 Sugar, Sugar Everywhere

Substitutes for refined sugar – raw sugar, stevia, not brown sugar which is white sugar with molasses mixed inAvailable at health food stores

Chapter 3 The Hidden Dangers Of White Flour

Whole grain flours such as spelt, whole wheat
Available at health food stores

Chapter 4 Salt – Just How Bad Is It?

Selina Naturally original and flavored salts, celery, smoked, rosemary, toasted sesame, toasted garlic
wwwselinanuaturally.com
1-800-867-7258
Can purchase direct from company

Chapter 6 Caffeine – The Mean Bean

Coffee substitute – Teeccino

www.teeccino.com

1-800-498-3434

Can purchase directly from company, Whole Foods Market or health food stores

Chapter 7 Enzymes – The Key To Life

Medizym Systemic Enzyme Formula

Nattokinase

www.naturally.com

1-800-899-4499

Megazymes (enzyme for digestion)

www.megafood.com

1-800-848-2542

Digestin (enzyme for digestion)

Progressive Labs

www.progressivelabs.com

1-800-527-9512

Can purchase direct from company

20% discount upon mention of this book

Chapter 8 Water

Pure and Secure
www.mypurewater.com
1-800-875-5915
Company is offering a factory direct price with an additional 10% discount upon mention of this book
Stainless steel is my preferred recommendation

Chapter 11 Joan's Picks

The items mentioned in this chapter can be purchased at health food stores, Whole Foods supermarkets and possibly some other elite supermarkets.

Chapter 12 Ailments and Diseases

Please refer to other chapters in this Reference Guide for the complete contact information for the various companies if not already mentioned.

Accelerated Aging – Omega-3 fatty acids (krill oil)
Gonado-F ovarian glandular for women by Progressive Labs and Nutricology, also Female Caps by Solaray
Orchic glandular for men by Progressive Labs

Alcoholism –Kudzu herb for cravings, milk thistle and dandelion for liver restoration and St. John's Wort for depression

Allergies – Liver Gallbladder extract by Quantum Herbals
Intestinal Cleansing Formula also by Quantum Herbals
Magnesium by MegaFood for chocolate cravings

Alzheimers – Nattokinase by Naturally VItamins
B, C, and E vitamins by MegaFood
ginko and antioxidants

Arthritis/Joint Inflammation - Collagen JS by Pure Encapsulations (1000 mg. chicken cartilage per 2 capsules)
Glucosamine Chondroitin by Pure Encapsulation
Medizym by Naturallly Vitamins
Omega 3 & 6 fatty acids

Asthma - Clear Lungs by Ridgecrest Herbals (Red Label)
Lung glandular by Nutricology

Atherosclerosis
Niacin – no flush type

Autism – stem cell research underway

Autoimmune Disease – a doctor of natural remedies to deal with the imbalance in the immune system

Blood Pressure – pomegranate
Nattokinase enzyme by Naturally Vitamins

Cancer – distilled water

No white flour, no white sugar

Medizym Systemic Enzyme Formula by Naturally Vitamins

Female cancers only – progesterone cream by Organic Excellence

Cholesterol – red yeast rice with CoQ10 by Solaray

Nattokinase by Naturally Vitamins

Guggul lipids

Beta glucan supplement

Common cold – Oil Of Oregano by North American Herb and Spice

Cod liver oil

Depression - B complex vitamins by MegaFood

St John's Wort herb

Omega-3 fatty acids (krill oil)

Diabetes – pancreas glandular by Progressive Labs or Nutricology

No refined sugar or refined white flour

CLA supplement

GTF chromium supplement

Diarrhea – homeopathic remedy Podophyllum

Epilepsy – magnesium by MegaFood may be helpful but a doctor's supervision is necessary

No alcohol, caffeine,

B complex vitamins by MegaFood

D vitamins by MegaFood

Omega-3 fatty acids (krill oil)

Eyesight – cod liver oil

Eye exercises

Opthamologist or optometrist who will step down your prescription lenses in conjunction with eye exercises

Essential fatty acids

Natural full spectrum lighting by Ott Lighting

Heart Health – omega-3 fatty acids (krill oil)

CoQ10 in ubiquinol form

Hearing – ear candling usually done by a massage therapist

Hiccups – please see Chapter 12 for detailed instructions

HIV – Lomatium Isolate by Eclectic (WITH alcohol)

Indigestion – Megazymes digestive enzymes by MegaFood

Probiotic supplement by Intestinal Care By Ethical Nutrients on an empty stomach, comes in capsules and powder, the powder is more economical

Reduce consumption of heavy proteins

Insomnia – Deep Sleep by Herbs, Etc.

More time outdoors

Exercise is very helpful

Natural full spectrum lighting by Ott Lighting

Too many microwave towers near your home

www.antennasearch.com

Intestinal Poisons – Intestinal Cleanser by Quantum Herbals

Kidney Problems – Selina Natural Salts (in moderation)
Distilled water
Kidney glandular from Progressive Labs Or Nutricology

Liver Problelms – cutting down on red meat
Liver Gallbladder Extract by Quantum Herbals
Eliminating alcohol, fried foods and fatty foods
Eliminating all unnecessary medications

Memory – DNA complex
Phosphatidyl serine DHA
Mental Sharp by Pure Encapsulations
Krill oil
Check for mold in the home

Menopause – please see chapter For Women Only

Migraine Headaches – Liver Gallbladder Extract by Quantum Herbals
Eliminate excess medication (not necessary prescriptions)
Improve diet

Osteoporosis – progesterone cream by Organic Excellence (women only)
Megazymes Digestive Enzymes by MegaFood
Cod liver oil
Calcium Magnesium Complex by Mega Food
Extra Magnesium tablet to balance calcium magnesium ratio to 1:1 instead of 2:1

Parasites – FOOD GRADE diatomaceous earth powder. Warning – this powder should not be inhaled

Prostate Problems – saw palmetto herb

Skin Disorders – Intestinal Cleansing Formula by Quantum Herbals

Skin Infections – topical ointment Ichthammol Ointment 20% by Goldline. This is not to be used in the mouth, ears, nose, or throat. For external use only

Transplants – glandular that corresponds to the ailing organ e.g. kidney glandular for kidney problems

Tumors – Medizym Systemic Enzyme Formula by Naturally Vitamins (the one with the enteric coating) not to be confused with the digestive enzyme. This MUST be taken on a totally empty stomach with no food for at least 45 minutes afterward.
Medizymes Digestive Enzymes taken with meals
Natural diet

Ulcers – Gastro Pro by Progressive Labs

Chapter 13 Glandular Therapy

Progressive Labs
www.progressivelabs.com
1-800-527-9512
Can purchase direct from company
20% discount upon mention of this book

Nutricology
www.nutricologly.com
1-800-545-9960

Solaray
Female Caps (ovarian glandular)
www.nutraceutical.com
Can purchase from health food stores Company does not sell direct to consumers

Chapter 14 Weight Gain/Loss

Norwegian Cod Liver Oil
Sold at health food stores

Quantum Herbals Liver Gallbladder Formula (tincture)
Quantum Herbals Intestinal Cleanser
www.quantumherbalproducts.com
1-845-246-1344
Can purchase direct from company or health food stores (may have to be a special order)

Pancreas glandular
www.progressivelabs.com
1-800-527-9512
Can purchase direct from company
20% discount upon mention of this book

www.nutricology.com
1-800-545-9960
Can purchase direct from company

GTF Chromium
www.megafood.com
1-800-848-2542
Can purchase from health food stores. Company does not sell direct to consumers

Chapter 16 Vitamins Anyone?

MegaFood

Optimum Foods (multivitam)

Vitamin D3

Calcium, Magnesium, Potassium

Magnesium

Chapter 17 For Women Only

Progesterone Cream

www.organicexcellenc.com

1-800-611-8331

See the link on my website joanyork.com

Gonado-F Ovarian Glandular

www.progressivelabs.com

1-800-527-9512

Can purchase direct from company

20% discount upon mention of this book

Solaray Female Caps Ovarian Glandular

www.nutraceutical.com

Can purchase from health food stores Company does not sell direct to consumers

Chapter 18 Pregnancy

Baby and Me (prenatal)
Baby and Me Herb-Free
www.megafood.com
1-800-848-2542
Can purchase from health food stores

Chapter 19 For Men Only

Anrdrozyme Orchic Glandular
www.progressivelabs,com
1-800-527-9512
Can purchase direct from company
20% discount upon mention of this book

Chapter 20 Getting Rid Of Pain The Natural Way

Pure Encapsulations
Collagen JS
Glucosomine Chrondroitin
www.purecaps.com
1-800-753-2277
Sold by health care professionals (chiropractors, registered nurses, naturo-
paths, registered dieticians)

Liver Gallbladder Formular (for migraines or headaches)
www.quantumherbalproducts.com
1-845-246-1344
Can purchase from health food stores or directly from the company

Chapter 21 Dental Secrets

Biocomp Labs
biocomplabs.com
1-719-548-1600

Natural Dentist mouthwash and toothpaste
www.thenaturaldentist.com
1-800-615-6895

Chapter 28 Indoor Pollution

Air filters that do not produce ozone
Gas fireplaces that are sealed and vented (excellent source of heat)
Biokleen household products
1-800-477-0188
www.biokleenhome.com
Can purchase direct from company

Chapter 30 Relieving Stress By Being Prepared

Solar generator
Water Distiller
Greenhouse

Chapter 37 Save Our Pets

Pet Guard wet and dry cat and dog food (mostly organic)

www.petguard.com

1-800-874-3221

Sold at Whole Foods Markets, Agway, and health food stores

Other Books By Joan York, B.S.

The Calendar Lies, Believe Your Eyes

Alternative Health Remedies For Cats

Alternative Health Remedies For Dogs

joanyork.com

Bibliography

Alkalize Or Die, Dr. Theodore A. Baroody

Caffeine Blues, Stephen Cherniske, M.S.

Enzyme Nutrition, Dr. Edward Howell

Google

Journal of Immunity

www.ingramcontent.com/pod-product-compliance
Lightning Source LLC
Chambersburg PA
CBHW081822280526
45789CB00007B/2299